# Atlas of
# DENTAL
# RADIOGRAPHY
## in Dogs and Cats

# Atlas of
# DENTAL
# RADIOGRAPHY
## in Dogs and Cats

**Gregg A. DuPont,** DVM
Fellow Academy of Veterinary Dentistry
Diplomate American Veterinary Dental College
Shoreline Veterinary Dental Clinic
Seattle, Washington

**Linda J. DeBowes,** DVM, MS
Diplomate American College of Veterinary Internal
Medicine (Small Animal)
Diplomate American Veterinary Dental College
Shoreline Veterinary Dental Clinic
Seattle, Washington

*with 837 illustrations*

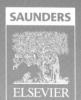

SAUNDERS
ELSEVIER

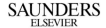

11830 Westline Industrial Drive
St. Louis, Missouri 63146

ATLAS OF DENTAL RADIOGRAPHY IN DOGS AND CATS

ISBN-13: 978-1-4160-3386-8
ISBN-10: 1-4160-3386-6

**Library of Congress Cataloging-in-Publication Data**

DuPont, Gregg A.
   Atlas of dental radiography in dogs and cats : a practical guide to techniques and interpretation / Gregg A. DuPont, Linda J. DeBowes ; with 837 illustrations. -- 1st ed.
       p. ; cm.
       Includes bibliographical references and index.
   ISBN-13: 978-1-4160-3386-8 (hardcover : alk. paper)
   ISBN-10: 1-4160-3386-6 (hardcover : alk. paper)
   1. Dogs--Diseases--Atlases. 2. Cats--Diseases--Atlases. 3. Dogs--Anatomy--Atlases. 4. Cats--Anatomy--Atlases. 5. Veterinary dentistry. 6. Veterinary radiology--Atlases. I. DeBowes, Linda J. II. Title.
   [DNLM: 1. Radiography, Dental--veterinary--Atlases. 2. Cats--anatomy & histology--Atlases. 3. Dogs--anatomy & histology--Atlases. 4. Mouth Diseases--radiography--Atlases. 5. Mouth Diseases--veterinary--Atlases. 6. Tooth Diseases--radiography--Atlases. 7. Tooth Diseases--veterinary--Atlases. SF 867 D938a 2009]
   SF992.M68D87 2009
   636.7'0897607572--dc22

                                                         2008009535

ISBN-13: 978-1-4160-3386-8
ISBN-10: 1-4160-3386-6

*Vice President and Publisher:* Linda Duncan
*Senior Acquisitions Editor:* Anthony Winkel
*Developmental Editor:* Maureen Slaten
*Publishing Services Manager:* Julie Eddy
*Senior Project Manager:* Celeste Clingan
*Design Direction:* Renee Duenow

Printed in China

Last digit is the print number:   9  8  7  6  5  4  3  2

## DEDICATION

*This book is dedicated to*
*the many giants in the field of veterinary dentistry*
*who preceded us and shared their knowledge and expertise,*
*and to those around us who are rapidly becoming the giants of tomorrow.*

*Also to the concept that while black and white may be the easiest to recognize,*
*the most important information is often found in the shades of gray.*

**Linda J. DeBowes and Gregg A. DuPont**

Veterinary students and professionals receive education and training in radiography of the skeletal and soft tissues in general, but very little training and experience reading dental and oral radiographs. Positioning the patient, the x-ray tube, and the film or sensor for intraoral radiography can be challenging because of anatomical and spatial limitations of the oral cavity, and the radiographic images can be difficult to interpret because of the regional anatomical complexities. Radiographic interpretation of normal oral anatomy can be misleading, confusing, and frustrating because multiple bone-dense structures and air-dense structures superimpose on the anatomy one actually wants to evaluate. Add some interesting pathology and the picture becomes even murkier.

Veterinary dentistry is a visual field. Most diagnoses are made by either direct observation of the oral cavity or by evaluation of radiographic images. Visual diagnostic accuracy depends both on the viewer's ability to perceive the problem and ability to interpret what is perceived. The ability to perceive radiographic anatomy and pathology requires good technique and good quality radiographs. The ability to interpret what is perceived is subject to the interpreter's ability, experience, and information. In preparing this textbook, pictures and visuals are maximized to show anatomy and pathology far better than our words. The purpose of the textbook is to help veterinarians and students improve their diagnostic accuracy and to become confident when identifying which structures and lesions are represented by the plethora of opacities and lucencies commonly seen on dental radiographs. These findings include normal things that appear normal, normal tissues that appear abnormal, and some of the abnormalities and disease processes commonly encountered in dogs and cats.

Our goal is to provide practical and easily accessible information that will add to your enjoyment of caring for the dental and oral health of your patients. We hope that you find the textbook helpful in your studies and your clinical practices.

*Linda J. DeBowes and Gregg A. DuPont*

# ACKNOWLEDGMENTS

Compiling a textbook requires a considerable amount of time and work. But when the topic is close to one's heart, it is a labor of love that seems more like an enjoyable, but demanding, hobby. The authors share their specialty practice, their devotion and immersion in veterinary dentistry, and their lives with each other. They bring their individual perspectives and experiences together to bring this book to you.

We would like to sincerely thank the many people who helped with the process by sharing information from their areas of expertise. Dr. Charles Root, DVM, MS, Diplomate ACVR, provided the CT studies of a normal dog and cat skull from which images were used to clarify the three-dimenionsal relationships of the structures that are imaged on dental and oral radiographs. Dr. Robert W. Kramer, DVM, Diplomate ACVR, generously shared his insights and information in the field of radiology, as did Dr. Donald E. Thrall, DVM, PhD, Diplomate ACVR, who kindly provided answers to numerous questions regarding accurate use of terminology.

We would also like to thank Dana Smith LVT and Lori Davis, our invaluable employees. They never complained (that we know of) throughout long months of retrieving records and data, and putting up with our "extracurricular" project.

Thanks also to Elsevier for identifying a need and for bringing this textbook to veterinary students and professionals. The company's ongoing commitment to providing high quality literature for health care professionals and ability to facilitate the process were essential. Working with Elsevier's veterinary Acquisitions Editor Dr. Anthony Winkel, Senior Project Manager Celeste Clingan, and Developmental Editor Maureen Slaten was a pleasure throughout the process.

Finally, we would like to acknowledge the contribution of the Pacific Northwest Coast beaches of the Olympic Peninsula. The setting provided encouragement, atmosphere, and key changes of venue to help us stay on task to create the best possible textbook for the readers.

*Linda J. DeBowes and Gregg A. DuPont*

# CONTENTS

Atlas of
# DENTAL
# RADIOGRAPHY
in Dogs and Cats

# Introduction to Dental Radiography

## Veterinary Dental Radiology

Dental and oral diseases, many of which cause discomfort and inflammation, are common in dogs and cats. These patients present a diagnostic challenge because they often show no outward sign of their discomfort. Furthermore, many of the methods that assist diagnosis in human patients, such as identification and localization of discomfort, thermal and electrical pulp testing, and local anesthesia testing, are not helpful in animal patients. In addition to these obstacles, most of the pathology-related tissues are below the gingival margin, hidden from direct visualization. So while radiography is a narrow method of adding additional information to that which we get during a physical examination, in the oral cavity it is a tremendously important one. In addition to diagnosing problems, dental and oral radiographs also provide critical information for treatment planning, treatment evaluation, and treatment success.

The information on radiographic images must be carefully considered during interpretation. Radiographic opacities and lucencies can be unreliable at best, and outright misleading at worst. Even among experts, there is large interobserver variation in the interpretation of dental radiographs. It has been shown that dentists significantly improved their diagnostic accuracy in finding radiographically visible features when they were given reference images with which to compare their radiographs. This book provides a readily available collection of reference dental and oral radiographic images, both of normal anatomy and of many of the pathological processes commonly found in dogs and cats.

## Basics of Radiographic Principles

The basic principles of dental and oral radiography are similar to those for general radiography—the goal is to achieve high-resolution (ability to visualize and differentiate small objects) images with sufficient contrast and gray scale to be able to see and identify the structures.

Radiographs are images of shadows that are cast by tissues and structures of varying radiopacity. Structures that absorb x-rays are radiopaque, and those that transmit them are radiolucent. The final radiograph merges all the structures in a three-dimensional area into a two-dimensional image. It could be considered similar to taking all the slices of a computed tomography study and printing them all on top of each other on a single page. The interpreter needs to mentally reexpand the flat image into its original multilayered size to help make sense of the information on it. Interpretation of radiographs is often facilitated by evaluating two views taken at 90-degree angles. Unfortunately, due to the adjacent anatomy, radiographs of teeth cannot be made along the mesiodistal (side-to-side) axis. Veterinary dental radiographs are mostly taken along the facial-oral axis. When superimposition of structures interferes with radiographic interpretation, oblique projection radiographs should also be made by changing the horizontal angulation (tube shift) while keeping the vertical angulation the same (see "bisecting angle" technique in Chapter 12).

Interpretation also follows the same rules as for general radiographs, including reading the entire film in a consistent manner and, if reading emulsion films, using a good source of illumination and magnification. An example of a good film-reading routine might be to first scan the entire film for an overall impression of the anatomy, looking for things that are present that should not be and for things that are not present but should be. Then evaluate each tooth crown, the pulp chambers, the root canals, the periodontal ligaments, the lamina dura for integrity, the trabecular bone, and finally the cortical bone.

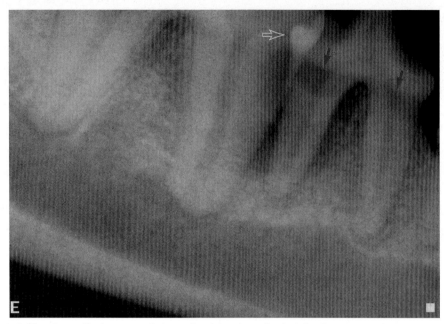

**FIGURE** 1-1 Structures that are radiolucent subtract radiodensity from superimposed structures, making them seem to disappear due to the summation effect. In this radiograph, the radiolucent regions on the roots of the fourth premolar and first molar teeth just below the crowns (*arrows*) are not defects in the teeth. They are caused by lack of overlying alveolar bone apically and enamel coronally. Conversely, when radiodense structures are superimposed across a relatively radiolucent structure, they can seem to appear from a void. In this case, the overlapping contact surfaces of the fourth premolar and first molar tooth allow visualization of the distal aspect of the premolar tooth (*open arrow*).

When evaluating a radiograph, always keep in mind the significance of multiple layers of overlapping structures. An important consequence of this is the "summation effect." The summation effect is the result of superimposed structures and tissues either adding to the radiopacity (addition) or subtracting from it (subtraction) depending on their relative radiopacities (Figure 1-1). Any object that can absorb x-rays and that is superimposed over bony structures will create the appearance of increased bone density in the area. Alternately, when an air-filled structure lies over bone, it will appear less dense. A second very important effect is the "tangential effect," in which two-dimensional details are diminished when they are perpendicular to the x-ray beam, while they are emphasized when they are parallel to the x-ray beam. This is true of both radiopaque and radiolucent structures. For example, the alveolus forms a white line where the bony plate parallels the x-ray beam and disappears where it is perpendicular to it. Similarly, a root fracture that makes a very black line when it is aligned parallel to the beam can completely disappear when perpendicular to the beam. A third effect involves the difficulty of localizing structures in the missing third dimension. Are they closer to the tube head, or closer to the film/sensor? This sometimes requires a second or third radiograph at different tube angle(s) to determine whether one structure is closer to, or farther from, the tube than a second close or overlapping structure (see "tube shift" in Chapter 12).

## Conventions for Textbook

The standard for veterinary gross anatomical nomenclature is the *Nomina Anatomica Veterinaria* (NAV). We have attempted to include many of these terms in italics in the normal sections. But even with the NAV and in today's world of shared informatics, agreement about correct terminology can be elusive. For example, the correct term for describing the surface of teeth that are facing outward away from the oral cavity is the "vestibular" surface. For the same surface of the maxilla (the bone that holds the canine, premolar, and molar teeth), the correct term is "facial," and for the mandible (the bone that holds all the lower teeth), the correct term is "buccal" for the premolar and molar area and "labial" for the incisor area. For this book, we have chosen to use nomenclature that is commonly accepted and in common use. For the above described surfaces, we used the terms "labial" when referring to the aboral surfaces of teeth or bones in the incisor and canine tooth areas and "buccal" when referring to the aboral surfaces of teeth or bones in the premolar and molar areas. We use the accepted dental nomenclature of "mesial" and "distal" to describe the directions toward the midline and away from the midline, respectively, when referring to teeth. When referring to bones and facial structures other than teeth, the terms "medial" and "lateral" would apply to the incisive area and "rostral" and "caudal" for the canine, premolar, and molar areas instead of "mesial" and "distal," respectively. In the same way, while "coronal" and "apical"

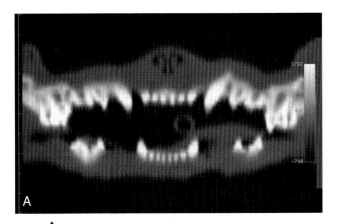

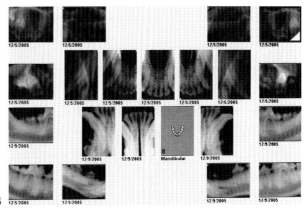

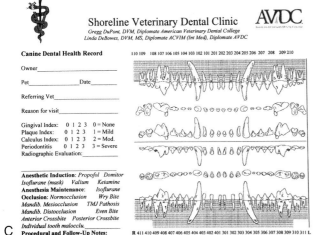

**FIGURE 1-2 Orientation of films for viewing. A,** Two-dimensional multiplanar reformat computed tomography image reconstruction simulates a panorama radiograph. This intuitive front-facial-view orientation of teeth is used for reading and storing radiographs. **(A,** *photograph courtesy of Dr. Robert W. Kramer.)* **B,** An example of a full mouth series of radiographs of a dog as stored in a digital radiography software template. The positions and orientations of the teeth in the radiographs approximate those on a panorama image. **C,** Section of a dental chart showing an anatomic depiction of the patient's teeth. The top row of teeth represents the labial and buccal surfaces of the maxillary teeth. The next row down represents the occlusal surfaces, and the third row from the top represents the palatal surfaces. The bottom row represents the labial and buccal surfaces of the mandibular arch. The next row up represents their occlusal surfaces, and the third row from the bottom represents their lingual surfaces.

are used to describe the vertical directions on the teeth, the terms "dorsal" and "ventral" are used for these dimensions on bones and nondental structures. The authors are aware of the fact that a structure on a brachycephalic animal could be physically "rostral" (i.e., toward the nose) but correctly termed "caudal" to another structure. But we use the term "rostral" because it is preferred to "anterior" by the NAV. Similarly, while the "permanent" dentition remains far less than permanent with the prevalence of severe periodontitis in today's pet population, we use the term "permanent" for the secondary dentition as directed by the NAV.

Nearly all the clinical dental radiographs were made using digital radiography (Schick Technologies CDR). The largest sensor size currently available is similar in size to a size 2 (periapical) dental film. Due to this size limitation, many of the radiographs used to demonstrate normal structures in the dog were made using conventional dental radiograph film exposed on size 4 (occlusal) F-speed film (Kodak Insight) and digitized with either a Nikon CoolPix 8400 or a CoolPix 995 camera. Clinical and specimen photographs were made using the CoolPix 995 camera.

This reference is designed primarily as a practical clinical tool to assist the user during interpretation of dental and oral radiographs of the dog and the cat. This is not intended to be a complete radiology text, but instead it concentrates on the

practical skills of making and interpreting radiographs. The first two sections show normal radiographic anatomy of the dog and cat. Each species section is divided into the adult maxillary arch, the adult mandibular arch, and the deciduous dentition. Radiographs depicting various lesions associated with a few common problems accompany the normal films to assist the practitioner in identifying both the normal and the abnormal anatomy; practitioners can quickly turn to the relevant anatomical location and compare their patient's film with the normal and abnormal examples shown.

Additional detail related to specific pathological processes follows the anatomical sections. These chapters are designed to help the practitioner or student understand the underlying processes that cause radiographic changes and to become familiar with a wider range of radiographic lesions related to each pathology. Finally, we discuss technique, a few basics of radiology, and equipment. These sections are meant to help the practitioner to identify artifacts and procedural problems, and are included both for individuals learning the basics of dental radiology and as a brush-up for the seasoned practitioner.

Throughout the text, radiographs are oriented as though the reader is looking at the patient (Figure 1-2). Maxillary teeth are oriented with the roots dorsal to the crowns, and mandibular teeth are oriented with the roots ventral to the

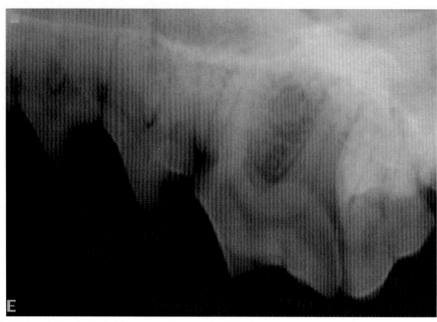

**FIGURE 1-3** Correct orientation for a radiograph of the left maxillary quadrant. Note that the roots are dorsal to the crowns. This identifies it as an upper tooth. The second and third premolar teeth are to the left of the fourth premolar, while the first molar tooth is to the right. This identifies it as the left quadrant.

crowns. A patient's right quadrants will show the molars to the left of the premolars, whereas the left quadrants will show the molars to the right of the premolars. This is the preferred viewing orientation for intraoral radiographs. It allows identification of individual teeth without the need to rely on film labels. For example, looking at the radiograph in Figure 1-3, the viewer can determine that it is a maxillary tooth due to the anatomy (presence of the nasal cavity and a three-root premolar). The roots are therefore oriented dorsally and the crown ventrally. With the convex "dot" toward the viewer, it can be seen that the third premolar is on the left, the fourth premolar is in the center, and the first molar is on the right. Therefore, this is the animal's left upper quadrant and the teeth are positioned as though you were looking at the patient's teeth in situ from the left side.

This orientation is achieved by viewing emulsion dental films that were exposed using intraoral technique with the convex side of the localization dot on the film toward the viewer and the concave side of the dot on the back of the film away from the viewer. It is also consistent with the default orientation of most digital radiography software when the sensor has been correctly placed in the patient's mouth for the selected template and position.

In Part Two, Radiographic Anatomy, a photograph of the relevant region of a skull will accompany many radiographs for clarification and to assist comprehension of the bony structures that contribute to the radiographic opacities. In many cases, we included mirror-image views of the same skull region viewed from the lingual or palatal surface. These are provided because the radiograph will record both surfaces (and everything between them) at once, and many surface features become valuable radiographic landmarks. Computed tomography scan images are included with selected radiographs to further clarify the relative three-dimensional positions and associations between structures that are depicted on the two-dimensional radiographic images.

## SUGGESTED READINGS

Pasler FA, Rateitschak KH, Wolf HF, eds: *Color Atlas of Dental Medicine—Radiology*, New York, 1993, Thieme Medical Publishers.

Stheeman SE, Mileman PA, van der Stelt PF: Diagnostic confidence and the accuracy of treatment decisions for radiopaque periapical lesions. *Int Endod J* 28:121-128, 1995.

Stheeman SE, Mileman PA, van Hof MA, van der Stelt PF: An approach to the development of decision support for diagnosing pathology from radiographs. *Dentomaxillofac Radiol* 24:38-42, 1995.

# CHAPTER 2

# Intraoral Radiographic Anatomy of the Dog

## THE NORMAL TOOTH

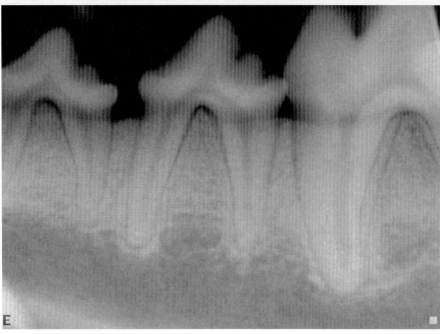

A  E

**FIGURE 2-1** Anatomy of the teeth and supporting structures. **A** and **B**, Radiograph of a left mandibular fourth premolar tooth. The third premolar tooth on the left and the first molar tooth on the right are partially imaged. **C** (*facing page bottom*), Prepared mandible sectioned to expose the internal anatomy. Intraoral radiographs clearly depict the anatomy of the teeth and the surrounding structures. Significant variability exists between individuals. A structure may be absent, be difficult to identify, or appear unusual in any particular individual radiograph. Note that the lamina dura, the white line around the root made by the compact bone of the alveolus (the tooth socket), is visible in some areas but absent in others. The bony plate of the alveolus is more apparent in areas where it is either parallel to the x-ray beam or is superimposed over other radiodense structures and much less apparent where it is perpendicular or tangential to the x-ray beam or is superimposed over radiolucent structures. There is significant variability in lamina dura density and presence between individuals. It is separated from the root by a radiolucent line that represents the periodontal ligament space. Enamel, the densest material in the tooth, covers the tooth crown and is also the most radiopaque material. It can appear as a narrow white line bordering the crown of a tooth, an effect that is enhanced on surfaces that are oriented more parallel to the axis of the x-ray beam. The enamel is often difficult or impossible to visualize on a radiograph because it is generally less than 0.6 mm thick. In many cases, the enamel only diffusely adds to the radiopacity of the crown. Dentin forms the majority of the mature tooth. It is less radiodense than enamel, but the roots appear to have a similar radiodensity to the enamel-covered crowns due to the superimposition of alveolar bone over the roots. The cervical area of the tooth, between the enamel of the crown and the alveolar bony margin, has neither enamel nor bone superimposed and is therefore less radiodense. This is referred to as "cervical burn-out" and should not be mistaken for caries or dental resorption. The bone of the alveolar margin should be relatively horizontal and positioned 1 to 2 mm apical to the cementoenamel junction. The interradicular marginal bone often has a slightly convex contour, filling the furcation area and closely approximating the contour of the furcation. In contrast, the interalveolar marginal bone (margin of septal bone) can have a horizontal, a slightly concave, or a slightly convex contour depending on the proximity of the adjacent roots and the particular region in the arch. The pulp cavity includes the root canal, found in the center of each root, and the pulp chamber in the crown. It appears radiographically as a comparatively radiolucent area within the tooth.

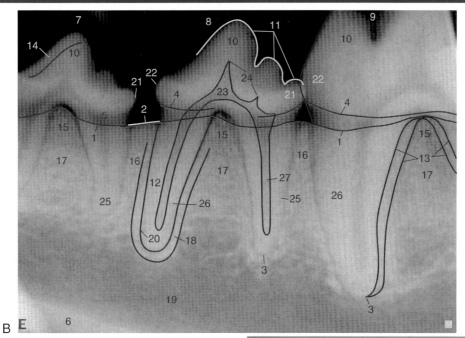

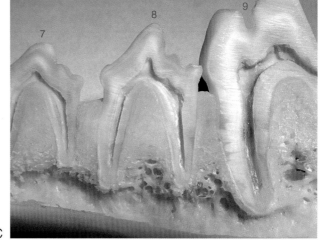

1. Alveolar margin (*margo alveolaris*)
2. Alveolar margin, interdental (*margo interalveolaris*)
3. Apex of root (*apex radicis dentis*)
4. Cementoenamel junction
5. Cervical area (*cervix dentis*)
6. Compact bone of ventral mandible (*margo ventralis*)
7. Third premolar tooth (*dentes premolares*)
8. Fourth premolar tooth (*dentes premolares*)
9. First molar tooth (*dentes molares*)
10. Crown (*corona dentis*)
11. Cusp (*cuspis dentis, tuburculum dentis*)
12. Dentin (*dentinum*)
13. Double shadow made by radicular groove
14. Enamel (*enamelum*)
15. Furcation area
16. Interalveolar septum (*septa interalveolaria*)
17. Interradicular alveolar septum (*septa interradicularia*)
18. Lamina dura—compact bone of alveolar wall
    (*alveoli dentales*)
19. Mandibular canal (*canalis mandibulae*)
20. Periodontal ligament space (*periodontium, articulatio dentoalveolaris*)
21. Proximal contact surface of tooth—distal
    (*facies contactus, facies distalis*)
22. Proximal contact surface of tooth—mesial
    (*facies contactus, facies mesialis*)
23. Pulp chamber (*cavum coronale dentis, pulpa coronalis*)
24. Pulp horn
25. Root—distal (*radix dentis*)
26. Root—mesial (*radix dentis*)
27. Root canal (*canalis radicis dentis, pulpa radicularis*)

## MAXILLARY INCISOR TEETH

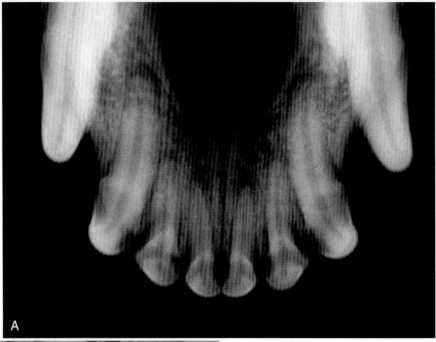

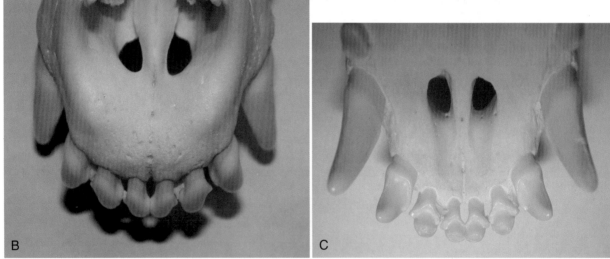

FIGURE 2-2 **Normal incisor teeth. A,** Radiograph of the incisor teeth and rostral maxillary region of a young adult dog. **B,** Dorsal view of prepared skull. **C,** Palatal (mirror) view of skull.

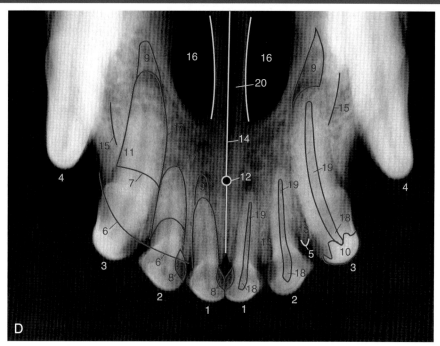

**FIGURE 2-2, cont'd  D,** Same radiograph as **A.** The crowns of the incisor teeth are foreshortened due to a projection angle that makes an image of the roots without elongation artifact (see Chapter 12).

1. First incisor tooth (*dentes incisivi*)
2. Second incisor tooth (*dentes incisivi*)
3. Third incisor tooth (*dentes incisivi*)
4. Canine tooth (*dentes canini*)
5. Alveolar margin, interdental (*margo interalveolaris*)
6. Alveolar margin, labial (*margo alveolaris*)
7. Alveolar margin, palatal (*margo alveolaris*)
8. Cervical burn-out
9. "Chevron" lucencies (see Figures 2-5 and 2-6)
10. Coronal enamel (accentuated due to tangential effect)
11. Dentin (*dentinum*)
12. Incisive canal (*canalis incisivus*) (varies in size and position and may be absent)
13. Interdental alveolar septum (*septa interalveolaria*)
14. Interincisive suture (*sutura interincisiva*)
15. Nasal process of the incisive bone (*processus nasalis, os incisivum*)
16. Palatine fissure (*fissura palatina*)
17. Periodontal ligament space (*periodontium, articulatio dentoalveolaris*)
18. Pulp chamber (*cavum coronale dentis, pulpa coronalis*)
19. Root canal (*canalis radicis dentis, pulpa radicularis*)
20. Vomer

# MAXILLARY INCISOR TEETH

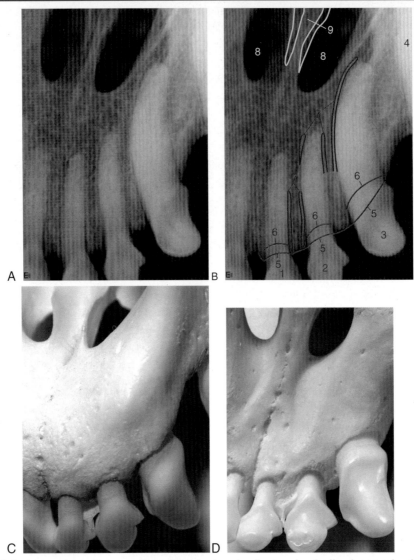

**FIGURE 2-3** In large dogs, the maxillary third incisor tooth can be better imaged using a more lateral projection angle. **A** and **B,** Radiograph of the left maxillary incisors. **C,** Labial view of a prepared skull. **D,** Palatal (mirror image) view of the skull. The left wing of the vomer is parallel to the x-ray beam and therefore more radiopaque than the right wing.

1. First incisor tooth
2. Second incisor tooth
3. Third incisor tooth
4. Canine tooth
5. Alveolar margin, labial
6. Alveolar margin, palatal
7. Lamina dura
8. Palatine fissures
9. Vomer

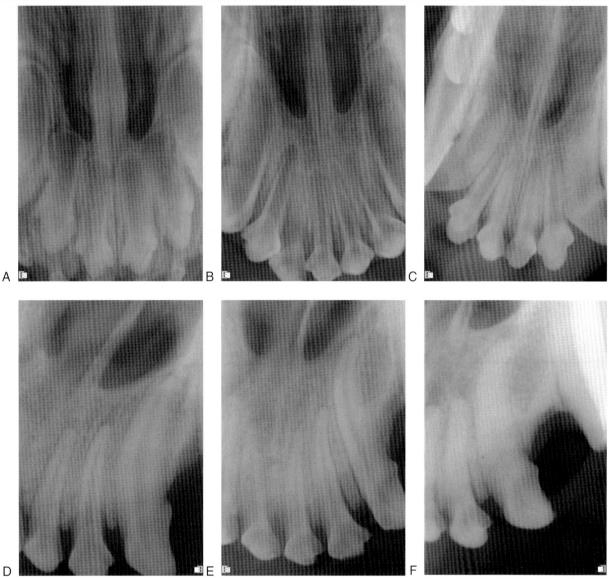

**FIGURE 2-4** Effect of aging on the size of the pulp chambers and root canals of incisor teeth. As teeth mature, secondary dentin is produced on the periphery of the pulp resulting in a progressively smaller pulp cavity with age. When the pulp experiences inflammation, dentin production can be accelerated resulting in a smaller pulp space compared to a healthy tooth. This can occur focally at the site of localized pulpitis. When it affects the entire pulp, the pulp appears more mature than normal. When a tooth pulp dies, maturation stops, making it appear less mature than normal (see Chapter 6). **A,** Three-month-old puppy. **B,** Five-month-old puppy. **C,** Eight-month-old puppy. **D,** Fifteen-month-old dog. **E,** Eighteen-month-old dog. **F,** Seven-year-old dog.

## MAXILLARY INCISOR TEETH

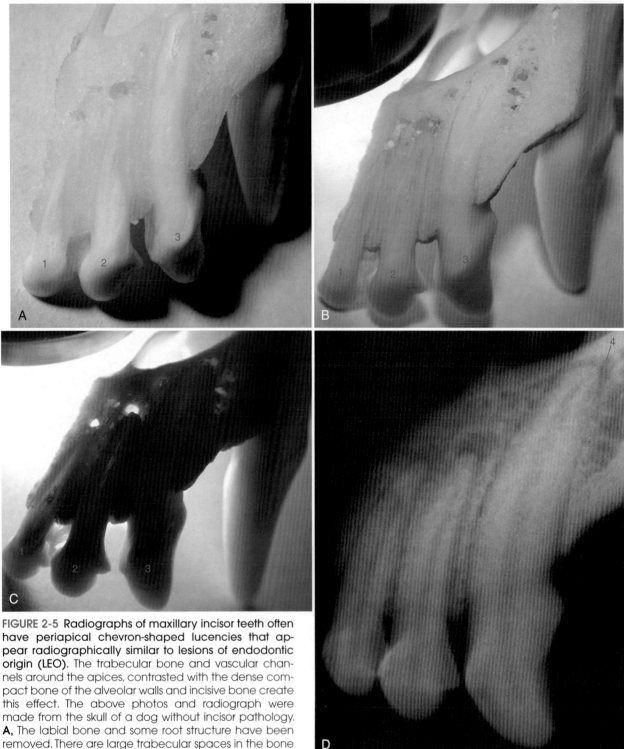

FIGURE 2-5 Radiographs of maxillary incisor teeth often have periapical chevron-shaped lucencies that appear radiographically similar to lesions of endodontic origin (LEO). The trabecular bone and vascular channels around the apices, contrasted with the dense compact bone of the alveolar walls and incisive bone create this effect. The above photos and radiograph were made from the skull of a dog without incisor pathology. **A,** The labial bone and some root structure have been removed. There are large trabecular spaces in the bone around the apices of all three incisor teeth. **B,** At a slightly more lateral angle and with rear illumination, one can view along a natural infrabony channel. **C,** With more intense rear illumination, the relatively thin bone density along the axis that an x-ray beam would travel becomes apparent. **D,** A radiograph of this skull preparation prior to removing any bone has typical chevron lucencies.

1. First incisor tooth
2. Second incisor tooth
3. Third incisor tooth
4. Normal radiographic lucencies that can mimic lesions of endodontic origin

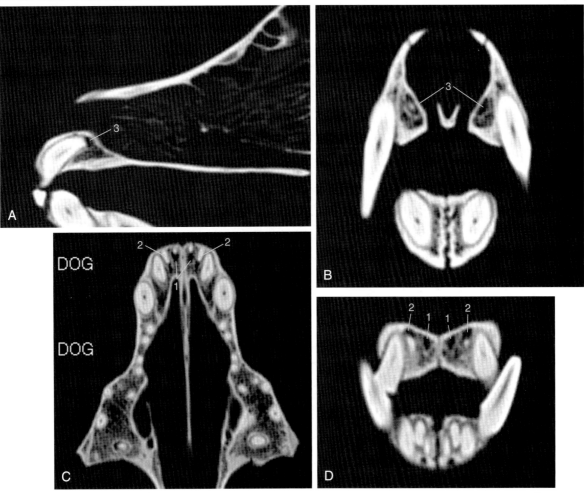

**FIGURE 2-6** In CT images, the periapical bone is characterized by large areas of hypoattenuation. These correspond to the region of decreased bone density around incisor root tips that result in radiolucent areas. **A,** Sagittal plane image at the level of the maxillary third incisor tooth. **B,** Transverse plane image at the level of the maxillary third incisor tooth apices. **C,** Dorsal plane image at the level of the first and second incisor tooth root apices. **D,** Transverse plane image at the level of the second incisor tooth root apices.

1. Apex and associated hypoattenuation of first incisor tooth
2. Apex and associated hypoattenuation of second incisor tooth
3. Apex and associated hypoattenuation of third incisor tooth

## MAXILLARY INCISOR TEETH

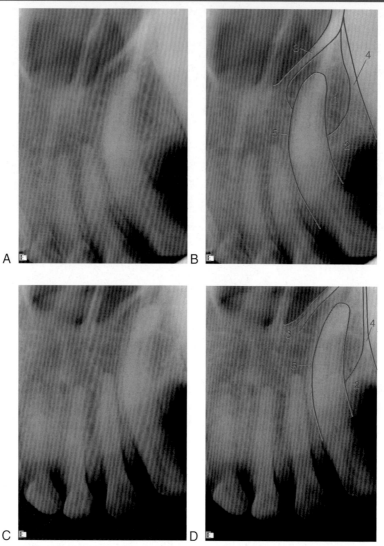

**FIGURE 2-7 Normal anatomy.** Summation effect can also mimic a lesion of endododontic origin when local radiodense structures are positioned in certain ways. **A** and **B,** The relative radiolucency around the apex of the left upper third incisor tooth is consistent with a LEO. However, the periodontal ligament space is intact around the apex. The appearance of an ovoid lucency is created by the normal compact bone of surrounding structures. **C** and **D,** The x-ray tube has been shifted from lateral to medial, providing a different view that more clearly displays the anatomy.

1. Area of relative radiolucency that can mimic a lesion of endodontic origin
2. Compact bone of alveolar margin of the incisive bone
3. Compact bone of the dorsal and nasal surface of the incisive bone
4. Compact bone of the mesial wall of the canine tooth alveolus
5. Periodontal ligament

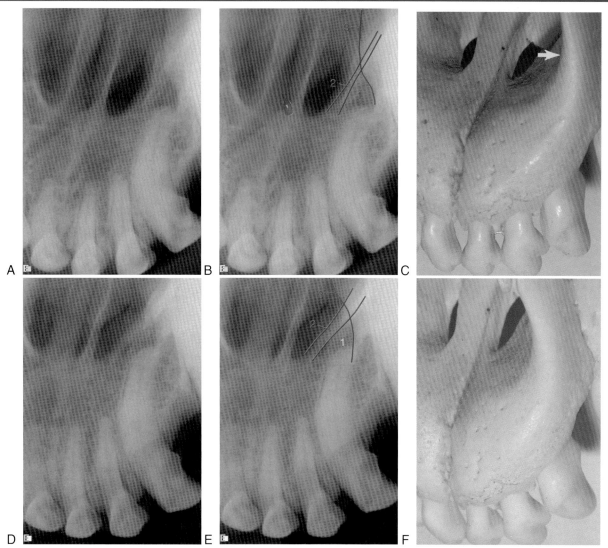

**FIGURE 2-8** Another example of summation effect mimicking a periapical lucency. **A** and **B,** Apparent radiolucency around the apex of the third incisor tooth. **C,** Skull showing how the nasal process of the incisive bone (*arrow*) makes a curved opacity that can appear to be the border of an endodontic lesion. **D** and **E,** The x-ray tube has been shifted to a more lateral position. The image of the incisive bone has shifted relative to the root apex, demonstrating that it is in a different plane from the root apex. The line of the incisive bone moved medially as the tube was shifted laterally indicating that the structure responsible for the linear opacity is labial to the tooth root (see Chapter 12). **F,** Skull showing how shifting the tube laterally moves the nasal process medially.

1. Area of relative radiolucency that can mimic a lesion of endodontic origin
2. Compact bone of the dorsal and nasal surface of the incisive bone
3. Nasal process of incisive bone

## MAXILLARY INCISOR TEETH

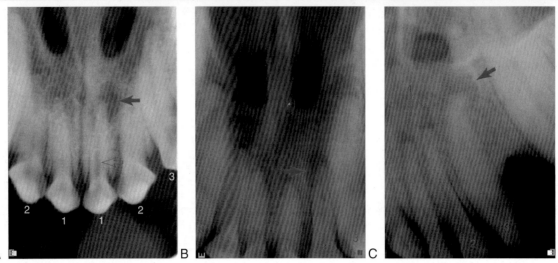

**FIGURE 2-9 True lesions of endodontic origin. A,** Periapical lucency of the bone around the apex of the left upper first incisor tooth (*arrow*). Note also the relative immature (wider) root canal and pulp chamber compared to the other incisor teeth (*open arrow*), consistent with pulp necrosis and arrested dentin production. **B,** Periapical lucency of the bone around the apex of the left upper second incisor tooth (*arrow*). **C,** Periapical lucency of the bone around the apex of the left upper third incisor tooth (*arrow*). Note the more circular shape compared to the chevron lucencies on the first and second incisor teeth. The radiopaque border is consistent with a chronic endodontic lesion (see Chapter 6).

1. First incisor tooth
2. Second incisor tooth
3. Third incisor tooth
4. Chevron lucency (normal)

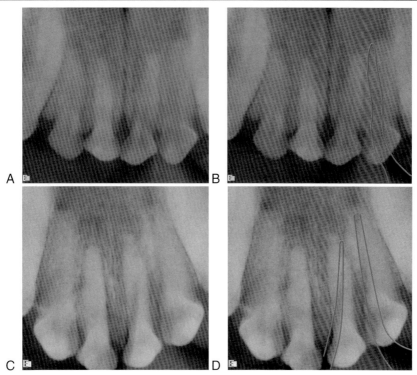

FIGURE 2-10 Superimposed hard and soft tissues can mimic oblique or vertical root fractures. **A,** Radiolucent lines where the nasal cartilage crosses the incisor roots. **B,** Same radiograph as **A** with cartilage outlined. **C,** Different soft tissue relationship. **D,** Same radiograph as **C.**

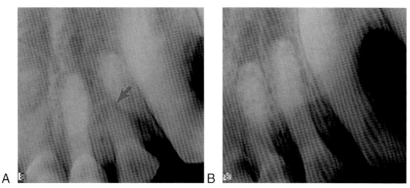

FIGURE 2-11 Superimposed structures mimic oblique root fracture. **A,** The left maxillary second incisor tooth has an oblique radiolucent line that appears to be a fractured root (*arrow*). However, the root canal space and the periodontal ligament spaces on both the mesial and distal sides remain perfectly linear with no disruption. **B,** A second view at a slightly different angle shows that the root is intact. Dental radiography is similar to general radiography in that two views provide more information than a single view.

## MAXILLARY INCISOR TEETH

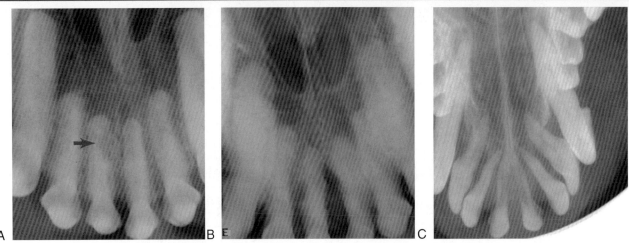

**FIGURE 2-12** Miscellaneous findings on radiographs of geriatric dogs. **A** and **B,** Cemental hyperplasia can occur unrelated to pathology or in the presence of pulpitis. It may often be a nonpathologic anomaly. It most commonly affects the apical third of the root creating a club-like appearance but can also affect the entire root. In **A,** there is also external root resorption (*arrow*). **C,** Horizontal bone loss of the alveolar margin in a geriatric dog with chronic periodontitis.

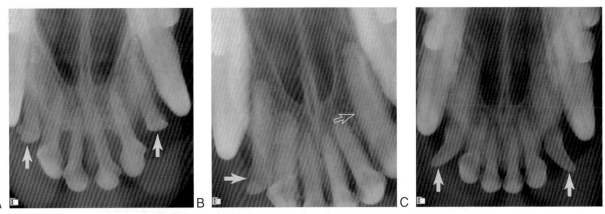

**FIGURE 2-13 A,** Persistent deciduous teeth. The first and second incisor teeth are permanent teeth. The third incisor teeth (*arrows*) are deciduous teeth with no succedaneous permanent teeth. The third incisor teeth should be larger than the first or second incisor teeth. **B,** In this dog, it is easier to see the difference; the right maxillary third incisor tooth (*arrow*) is a deciduous tooth, but the left maxillary third incisor tooth (*open arrow*) is a permanent tooth. **C,** This dog's permanent third incisor teeth (*arrows*) have the appearance of deciduous teeth due to rotation. The lateral view of the crowns makes them appear small. However, the roots are a normal size for permanent third incisor teeth.

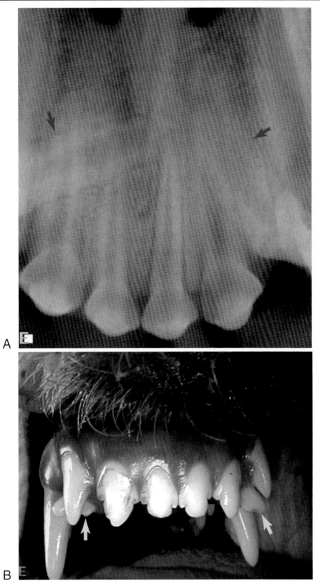

**FIGURE 2-14** Malpositioned supernumerary third incisors. **A,** Overlying root shadows (*arrows*) in an abnormal position (see Chapter 9). **B,** Clinical picture of the dog in **A.**

**CANINE TEETH**

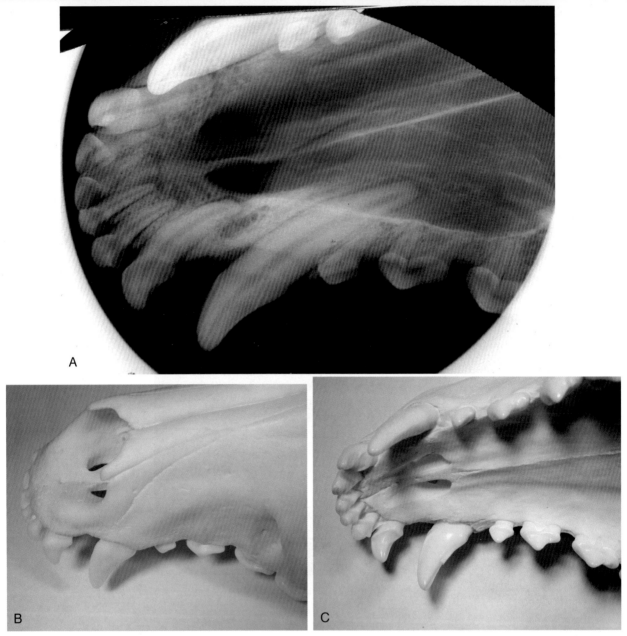

FIGURE 2-15 **Normal dog canine tooth. A,** Radiograph of the skull of a young dog showing the canine tooth and surrounding structures. **B,** Dorsal view of prepared skull. **C,** Ventral (mirror) view of skull.

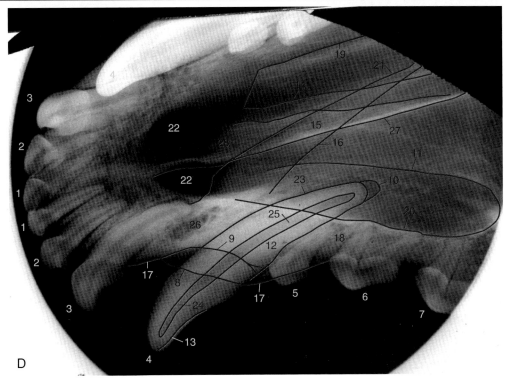

**FIGURE 2-15, cont'd  D,** Same radiograph as **A.**

1. First incisor tooth (*dentes incisivi*)
2. Second incisor tooth (*dentes incisivi*)
3. Third incisor tooth (*dentes incisivi*)
4. Canine tooth (*dentes canini*)
5. First premolar tooth (*dentes premolares*)
6. Second premolar tooth (*dentes premolares*)
7. Third premolar tooth (*dentes premolares*)
8. Alveolar margin, labial (vestibular) (*margo alveolaris*)
9. Alveolar margin, palatal (lingual) (*margo alveolaris*)
10. Chevron-shaped lucency
11. Conchal crest (*crista conchalis*)
12. Dentin (*dentinum*)
13. Enamel (*enamelum*)
14. Ethmoid crest (*crista ethmoidalis*)
15. Incisive bone, nasal process (*os incisivum, processus nasalis*)
16. Incisivomaxillary suture (*sutura incisivomaxillaris*)
17. Interalveolar margin (*margo interalveolaris*)
18. Interalveolar septum (*septa interalveolaria*)
19. Internasal suture (*sutura internasalis*)
20. Nasal surface of the alveolar process of the maxilla (*processus alveolaris*)
21. Nasoincisive suture (*sutura nasoincisiva*)
22. Palatine fissure (*fissura palatina*)
23. Periodontal ligament space (*periodontium, articulatio dentoalveolaris*)
24. Pulp chamber (*cavum coronale dentis, pulpa coronalis*)
25. Root canal (*canalis radicis dentis, pulpa radicularis*)
26. Trabecular bone (*substantia spongiosa ossium*)
27. Vomer—left wing (*ala vomeris*)
28. Vomer—right wing (*ala vomeris*)

**CANINE TEETH**

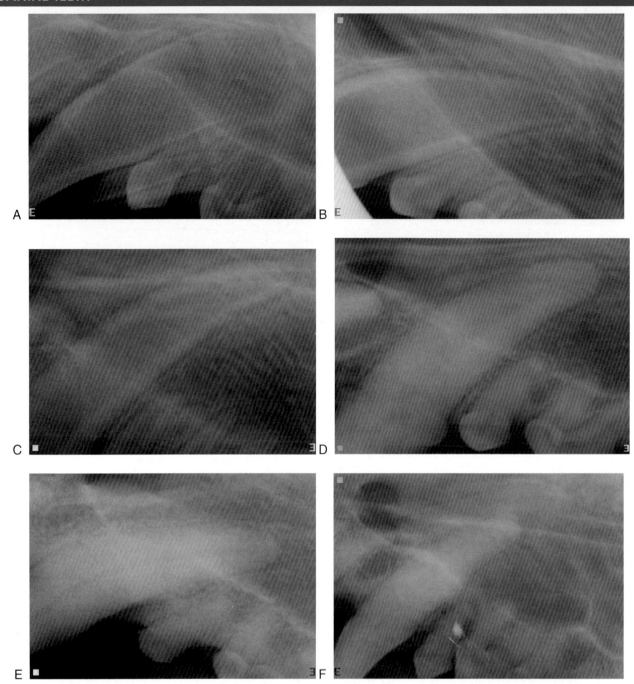

**FIGURE 2-16** Radiographs of canine teeth of different aged dogs shows the effect of age on size of the pulp chamber and root canal. **A,** Five-month-old Standard Poodle. **B,** Eight-month-old Bouvier. **C,** Eleven-month-old Labrador. **D,** Same dog as in **C** at 2 years of age. **E,** Nine-year-old Akita. **F,** Thirteen-year-old Terrier mix. The radiopaque spots are remnants of pumice polish.

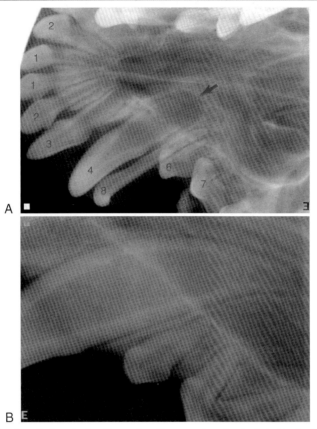

**FIGURE 2-17 Individual variation in tooth maturation and apical closure. A,** Radiograph from an 8-month-old Yorkshire Terrier. The apex is wide open with no apical constriction (*arrow*). Radiographs of small patients can include the entire canine tooth as well as surrounding anatomy, even on a size 2 film or digital sensor. This dog is missing the first premolar tooth and has a persistent deciduous canine tooth and a deciduous second premolar cap ready to exfoliate. **B,** Radiograph from a 9-month-old Bearded Collie. This tooth is significantly more mature than the tooth in **A** even though the dog is only 1 month older. The apex is already closed. The mesial root of the second premolar tooth is dilacerated at the apex (*open arrow*).

1. First incisor tooth
2. Second incisor tooth
3. Third incisor tooth
4. Canine tooth
5. First premolar tooth
6. Second premolar tooth
7. Third premolar tooth
8. Deciduous canine tooth
9. Deciduous second premolar tooth

## CANINE TEETH

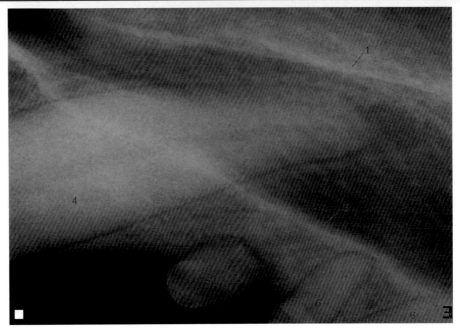

**FIGURE 2-18 Normal canine tooth with a periapical chevron shaped lucency similar to those seen on incisor teeth.** These lucencies extend apically from the apex and are sometimes quite large. They can be mistaken for lesions of endodontic origin. However, they are very regular in shape, extending the contour of the alveolus in a gently pointed arc rather than appearing as an expanded circular or irregular shape that is typical of endodontic lesions. With careful scrutiny, a periodontal ligament space and a faint lamina dura can often be seen closely approximating the root itself. This dog also has an anomalous first premolar tooth. A very prominent white line is made by the nasal surface of the alveolar process. This bony plate forms the ventrolateral wall of the nasal cavity, diagonally connecting the nasal surfaces of the palatal process (horizontal plate) and the body (vertical plate) of the maxilla. Its marked radiopacity is a result of its orientation parallel to the x-ray beam during bisecting angle technique radiographs of canine and premolar teeth. Further caudal this dorsal plate of the alveolar process forms the floor of the infraorbital canal. In the molar area it forms the floor of the pterygopalatine fossa.

1. Conchal crest and left wing of vomer
2. Chevron lucency
3. Nasal surface of the alveolar process of the maxilla
4. Canine tooth
5. First premolar tooth (anomalous)
6. Second premolar tooth

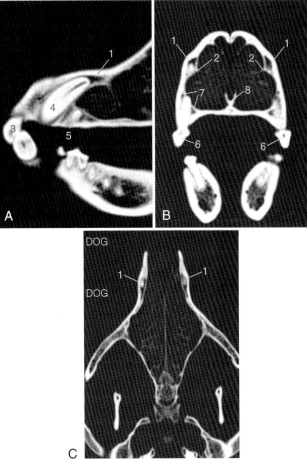

**FIGURE 2-19 CT scan images. A,** Sagittal plane. **B,** Transverse plane. **C,** Dorsal plane. The hypoattenuated areas around the apices of the canine teeth are caused by relatively less bone in an irregular cone shape. The borders are composed of the compact bone of the facial surface of the maxilla laterally and dorsally, and of the nasal surface of the maxilla medially and ventrally.

1. Area with no compact bone around root tip
2. Conchal crest
3. Third incisor tooth
4. Canine tooth roots
5. First premolar tooth
6. Second premolar tooth
7. Nasal surface of the alveolar process of the maxilla (*processus alveolaris*)
8. Vomer

## CANINE TEETH

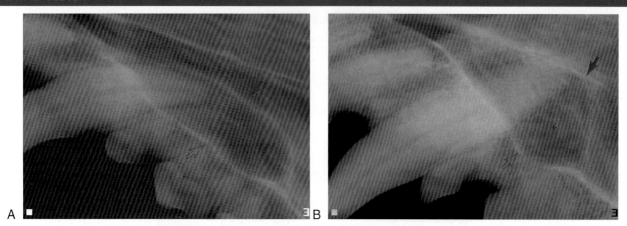

**FIGURE 2-20** The summation of multiple superimposed radiopaque and radiolucent structures can also mimic a lesion of endodontic origin (*asterisks*). **A** and **B** demonstrate the anatomic variability in appearance of the conchal crest (*arrow*) and nasal surface of the alveolar process (*open arrow*) in a long-nosed (**A**) and a short-nosed (**B**) dog.

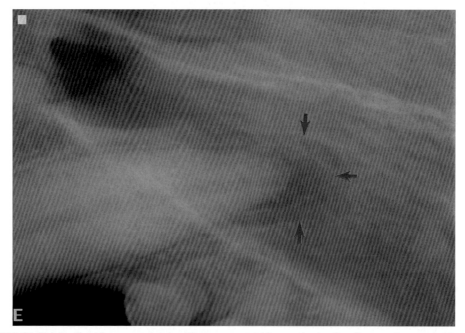

**FIGURE 2-21** This patient has a periapical lesion caused by endodontic disease (*arrows*). The lesion is not contiguous with normal anatomical structures.

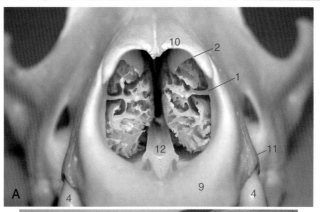

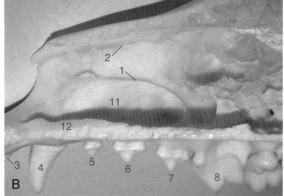

**FIGURE 2-22** Radiopaque structures on nasal surface of maxillary bones. **A,** Frontal view into the nasal aperture of a dog skull. The attachments of the middle and dorsal conchae to the nasal surface of the maxilla are visible. **B,** View of the nasal surface of the bones lining the nasal cavity. The conchae have been removed to reveal the contour of the conchal crest.

 1. Conchal crest
 2. Ethmoid crest
 3. Third incisor tooth
 4. Canine tooth
 5. First premolar tooth
 6. Second premolar tooth
 7. Third premolar tooth
 8. Fourth premolar tooth
 9. Incisive bone
10. Nasal bone
11. Maxilla
12. Vomer

## MAXILLARY PREMOLAR TEETH

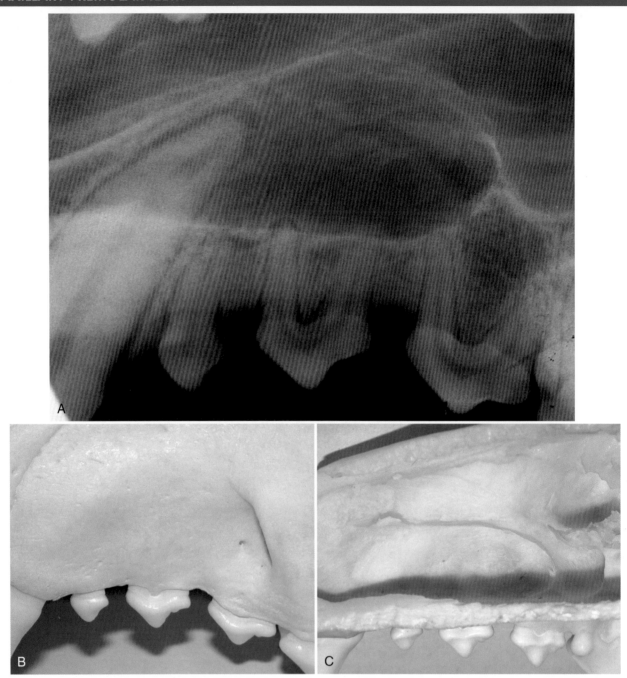

**FIGURE 2-23 Normal maxillary premolar teeth.** The facial and palatal region of the dog consists of 36 bones designed to provide a large surface area for the sense of smell and to hold the teeth. The premolar teeth are all within the alveolar process of the maxilla. However, radiographs of the premolar teeth may project through the nasal, frontal, palatine, and zygomatic bones. **A,** Radiograph of the left maxillary premolar region of a young dog. **B,** Buccal (vestibular) view of prepared skull. **C,** Nasal surface of maxilla.

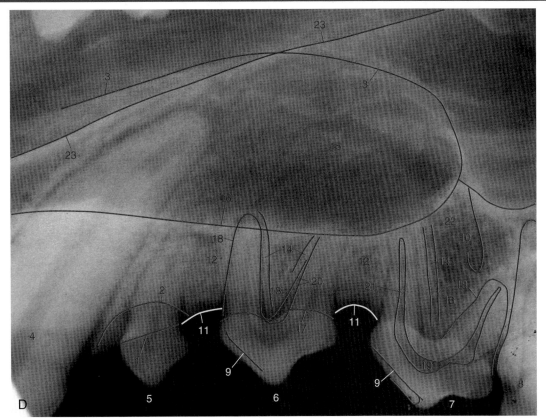

**FIGURE 2-23, cont'd D,** Same radiograph as **A.** Correct use of the bisecting angle technique makes an image with accurate root length. The apical anatomy, however, will be slightly enlarged due to an increased object-to-film distance at the apex.

1. Alveolar margin, buccal (*margo alveolaris*)
2. Alveolar margin, palatal (*margo alveolaris*)
3. Conchal crest (*crista conchalis*)
4. Canine tooth (*dentes canini*)
5. First premolar tooth (*dentes premolares*)
6. Second premolar tooth (*dentes premolares*)
7. Third premolar tooth (*dentes premolares*)
8. Fourth premolar tooth (*dentes premolares*)
9. Coronal enamel (*enamelum*)
10. Infraorbital foramen (*foramen infraorbitale*)
11. Interalveolar margin (*margo interalveolaris*)
12. Interdental alveolar septum (*septa interalveolaria*)
13. Interradicular bone (*septa interradicularia*)
14. Lamina dura—compact bone of alveolar wall (*alveoli dentales*)
15. Nasal cavity (*cavum nasi*)
16. Nasal surface of the alveolar process of the maxilla (*facies nasalis, processus alveolaris*)
17. Palatal marginal crown contour
18. Periodontal ligament space (*periodontium, articulatio dentoalveolaris*)
19. Pulp chamber (*cavum coronale dentis, pulpa coronalis*)
20. Radicular groove—double linear periodontal ligament lucencies
21. Root canal (*canalis radicis dentis, pulpa radicularis*)
22. Trabecular bone (*substantia spongiosa ossium*)
23. Vomer

## MAXILLARY PREMOLAR TEETH

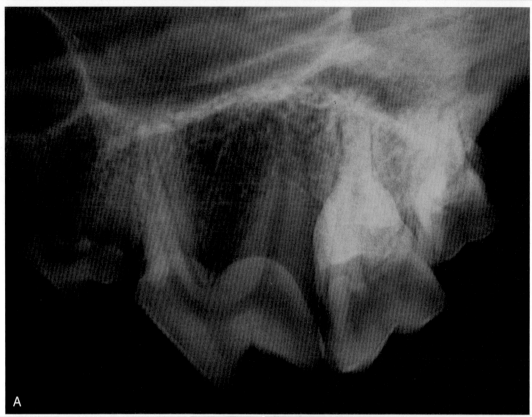

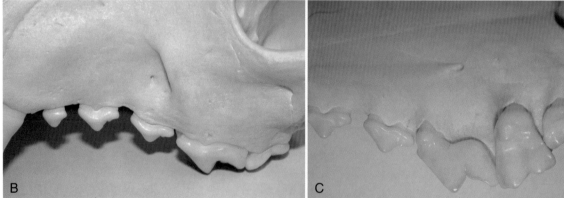

FIGURE 2-24 The maxillary fourth premolar tooth is often radiographed separately since it can be difficult to include all four premolar teeth on a single radiograph. **A,** Radiograph of a left maxillary fourth premolar tooth. The third premolar and the first and second molar teeth are also visible. **B,** Buccal view of a skull preparation. **C,** Palatal view (mirror image) of a skull preparation. **D** (*facing page top*), Same radiograph as **A. E** (*facing page middle left*), View of the nasal surface of the maxilla. The conchae have been removed. **F** (*facing page bottom right*), Transverse CT image at the level of the mesiobuccal and palatal roots of the fourth premolar helps to visualize how the dorsal plate of the alveolar process becomes the floor of the infraorbital canal.

1. Conchal crest (*crista conchalis*)
2. Distal root of fourth premolar tooth
3. Enamel (*enamelum*)
4. Infraorbital canal (*canalis infraorbitalis*)
5. Infraorbital foramen (*foramen infraorbitale*)
6. Interdental alveolar septum (*septa interradicularia*)
7. Third premolar tooth (*dentes premolares*)
8. Fourth premolar tooth (*dentes premolares*)
9. First molar tooth (*dentes molares*)
10. Second molar tooth (*dentes molares*)

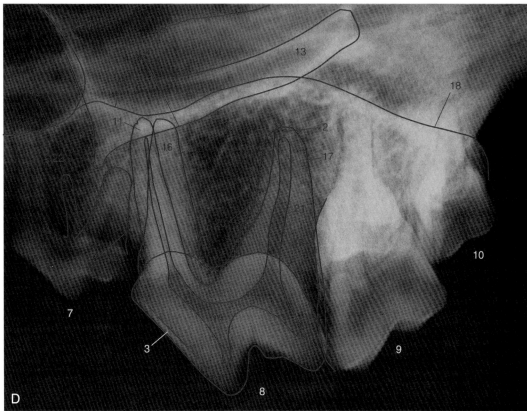

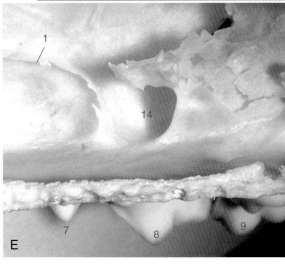

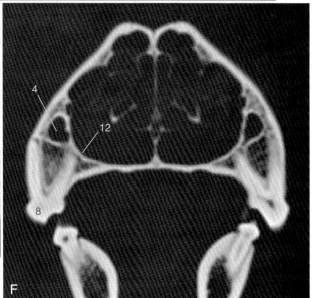

11. Mesiobuccal root of fourth premolar tooth
12. Nasal surface of the alveolar process of the maxilla (*processus alveolaris*)
13. Palatine canal (*canalis palatinus*)
14. Opening to the maxillary recess (*hiatus maxillaris*)
15. Palatal marginal enamel
16. Palatal root of fourth premolar tooth
17. Periodontal ligament space (*periodontium, articulatio dentoalveolaris*)
18. Pterygopalatine fossa, ventral surface (*fossa pterygopalatina*)
19. Pulp chamber (*cavum coronale dentis, pulpa coronalis*)
20. Radicular groove—double periodontal ligament spaces
21. Root canal (*canalis radicis dentis, pulpa radicularis*)
22. Supernumerary root
23. Trabecular bone (*substantia spongiosa ossium*)

## MAXILLARY PREMOLAR TEETH

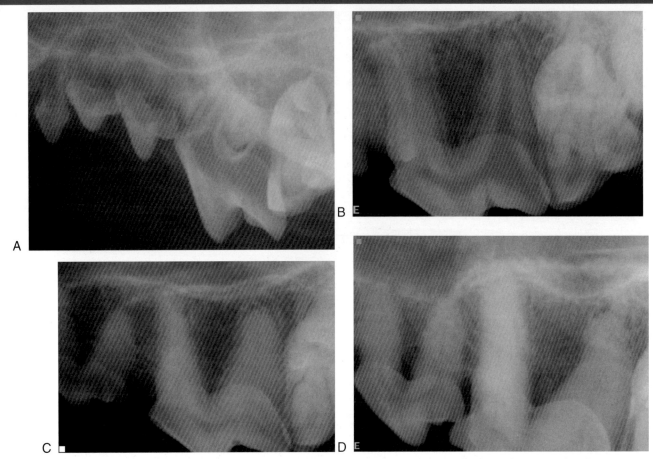

**FIGURE 2-25 The effect of age.** Dentin continues to be produced as the tooth matures causing the pulp chamber and root canal space to decrease in size. **A,** Seven-month-old Pomeranian. The apices are open. **B,** One-year-old Retriever. The apices are closed, but the pulp cavity (root canal spaces and pulp chamber) is large. **C,** Ten-year-old Belgian Sheepdog. The root canals and pulp chambers show marked attenuation. **D,** Fourteen-year-old Bassett Hound. The fourth premolar tooth demonstrates *pulp canal obliteration,* a radiographic term describing the inability to visualize the attenuated root canal space (see Chapter 6). This radiograph also demonstrates loss of the peri-odontal ligament space with the appearance of enlargement of the roots. These findings are consistent with cemental hyperplasia and possible root ankylosis.

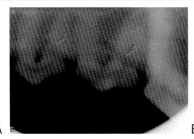 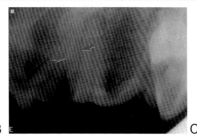 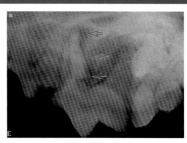

A   B   C

**FIGURE 2-26** Superimposed tissues crossing roots can mimic intraalveolar transverse and oblique root fractures. **A,** Oblique soft tissue shadows cross the roots of the normal second and third premolar teeth (*arrows*). Note that the shadows extend beyond the roots, and the periodontal ligament space and root canals are intact. **B,** The periodontal ligament of the palatal root of the fourth premolar tooth crosses the mesiobuccal root and the distal root of the third premolar to mimic oblique root fractures (*arrows*). The crown is badly fractured but the roots are intact. **C,** A true transverse fracture of the palatal root (*arrow*). The crown appeared normal. The periodontal ligament is not intact and has a marked step. The palatal and distal roots have periapical lucencies (*open arrows*).

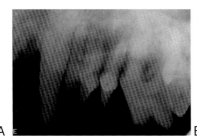 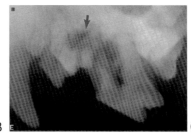 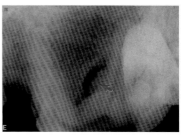

A   B   C

**FIGURE 2-27** Miscellaneous abnormalities. **A,** Crowded premolar teeth with severely rotated second and third premolar teeth (*asterisks*) in a brachycephalic dog. There is loss of septal and interradicular density indicating alveolar bone loss. These are common findings in areas affected with periodontitis (see Chapter 5). **B,** Severe crowding without rotation. Periapical radiolucency (*arrow*) indicates periodontal disease with secondary endodontic involvement (see Chapter 6). **C,** Calculus accumulation on the mesial aspect of the distal root of the left maxillary fourth premolar tooth with associated bone loss appears as a root surface radiopacity surrounded by a radiolucency (*arrow*).

## MAXILLARY PREMOLAR TEETH

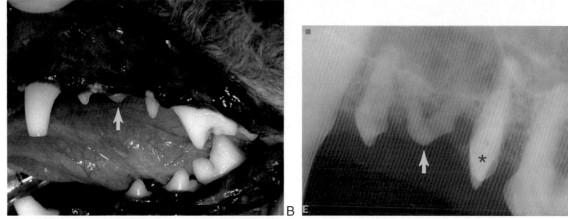

**FIGURE 2-28** Persistent deciduous maxillary second premolar tooth with no succedaneous permanent tooth. This is a relatively common abnormality in small-breed dogs. **A,** The second premolar tooth has a small clinical crown (*arrow*). **B,** A radiograph of this tooth shows a very small and relatively radiolucent second premolar tooth (*arrow*). Note also rotation of the third premolar tooth (*asterisk*). Summation effect of the two roots superimposed results in increased radiopacity.

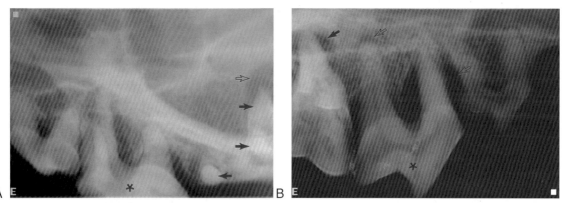

**FIGURE 2-29** Importance of reading the entire film. Both of these radiographs were made to evaluate periodontal disease with endodontic involvement of the fourth premolar teeth (*asterisks*). **A,** The molar teeth are gone but there are multiple persistent root fragments (*arrows*). There is a periapical lucency associated with the palatal root of the second molar (*open arrow*). **B,** The palatal root of the first molar tooth has a periapical lucency indicating endodontic disease (*arrow*). The fourth premolar tooth has a periodontal defect and an endodontic lesion (*open arrows*).

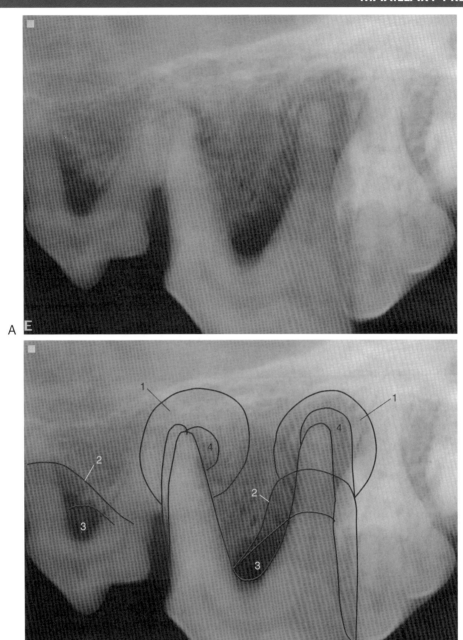

**FIGURE 2-30** Multiple radiographic findings.

1. Condensing osteitis indicating a chronic lesion.
2. Loss of buccal plate from periodontitis
3. Loss of both buccal and palatal bone in furcation
4. Periapical and periradicular lucencies consistent with lesions of endodontic origin

## MAXILLARY MOLAR TEETH

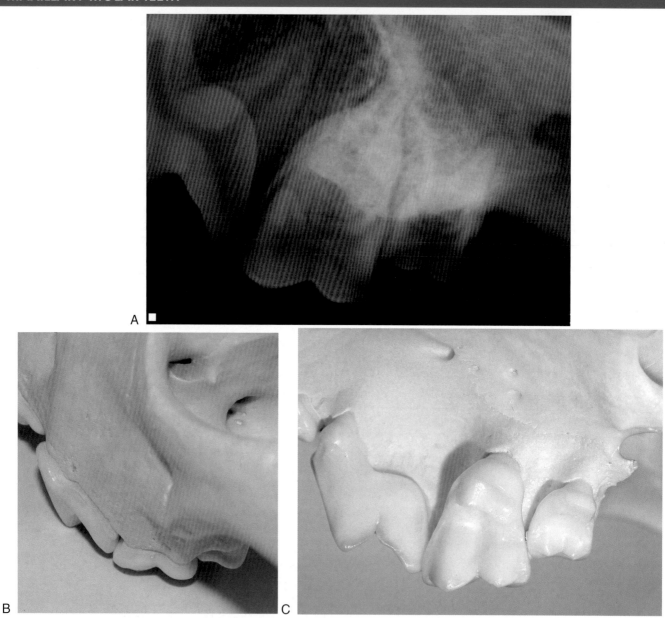

**FIGURE 2-31  Normal maxillary molar teeth.  A,** Radiograph of left maxillary molars. **B,** Buccal view of molar region of skull. **C,** Palatal view (mirror image) of molar region of skull.

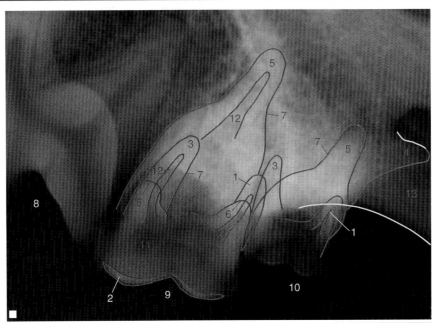

D

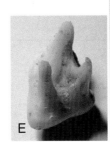

E

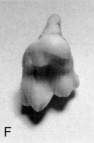

F

**FIGURE 2-31, cont'd  D,** Same radiograph as **A.** The occlusal enamel superimposed over the crown and the mesiobuccal and distal roots can mimic short roots. **E,** Extracted first molar tooth, buccal view. Bisecting angle technique makes the palatal root appear much longer than the other two roots. **F,** Extracted first molar tooth, palatal view. The two buccal roots are viewed through the crown on radiographs.

1. Distal root (*radix dentis*)
2. Enamel (*enamelum*)
3. Mesiobuccal root (*radix dentis*)
4. Pterygoid process of the maxilla (*processus pterygoideus*)
5. Palatal root (*radix dentis*)
6. Overlap of occlusal enamel, crown, and roots
7. Periodontal ligament/space (*periodontium, articulatio dentoalveolaris*)
8. Fourth premolar tooth (*dentes premolares*)
9. First molar tooth (*dentes molares*)
10. Second molar tooth (*dentes molares*)
11. Pulp chamber (*cavum coronale dentis, pulpa coronalis*)
12. Root canal (*canalis radicis dentis, pulpa radicularis*)
13. Zygomatic arch

## MAXILLARY MOLAR TEETH

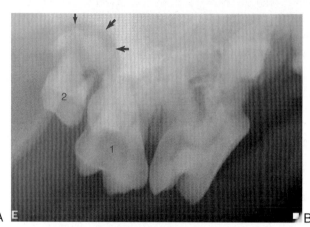
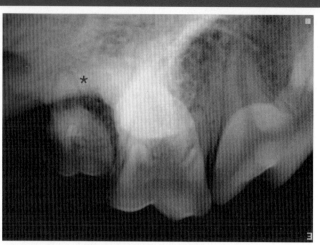

FIGURE 2-32 **A,** Normal radiolucency that can mimic a fracture of the maxillary tuberosity (*arrows*). **B,** Radiograph of a skull specimen using an angle and technique to reproduce the effect. This appearance is caused by summation effect (burn-out) below the radiodense zygomatic arch (*asterisk*). First molar (1), second molar (2).

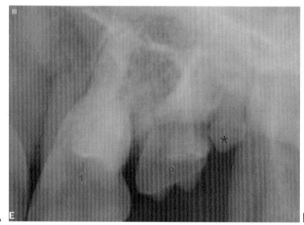
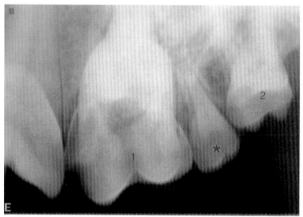

FIGURE 2-33 **Supernumerary molar teeth. A,** Bassett hound with a maxillary third molar tooth (*asterisk*). Dogs normally do not have maxillary third molar teeth. **B,** Dog with an abnormal and small supernumerary molar tooth (*asterisk*) between the first (1) and second (2) molar teeth (*arrow*).

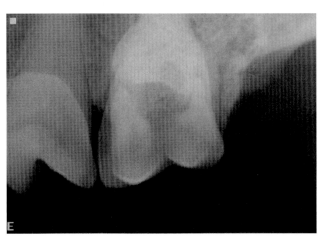

**FIGURE 2-34** Persistent mesiobuccal root fragment of the missing second molar tooth (*arrow*). This radiograph illustrates the importance of evaluating sites where teeth are missing and of reading the entire film.

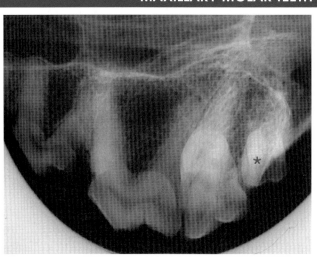

**FIGURE 2-35** Resorptive lesion (see Chapter 7). This radiograph was made to evaluate the fractured fourth premolar tooth. The roots of the second molar tooth (*asterisk*) are losing their radiodensity. This is consistent with one type of dental resorptive lesion.

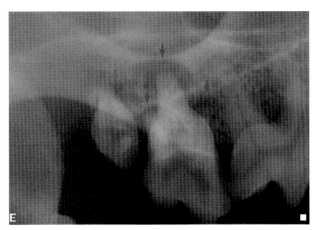

**FIGURE 2-36** Lesions of endodontic origin (see Chapter 6) appear as circular radiolucencies around all three root tips of the right maxillary first molar tooth (*arrows*) and the palatal root of the second molar tooth (*open arrow*).

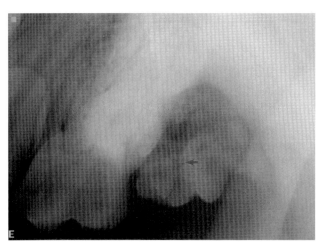

**FIGURE 2-37** Fractured crown of left maxillary second molar tooth (*arrow*). The first molar tooth is on the left, and the ramus of the mandible is to the right of the molars.

## MANDIBULAR INCISOR TEETH

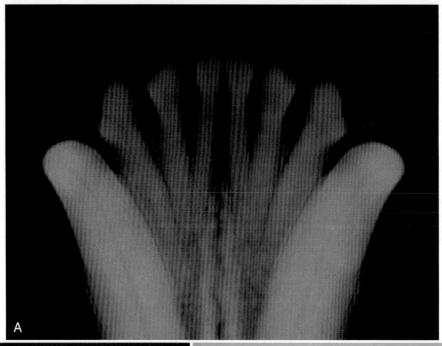

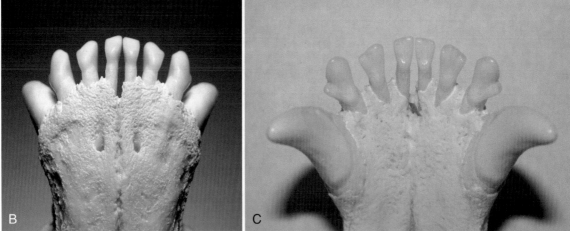

FIGURE 2-38  **Mandibular incisor teeth.** **A,** Radiograph of the incisor teeth and rostral mandibular region of a mature dog. **B,** Ventral view of rostral mandibles from a prepared skull. **C,** Dorsal (mirror image) view of the rostral mandibles.

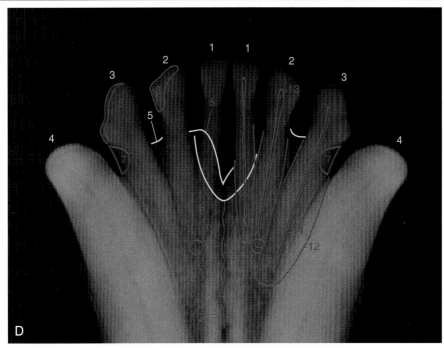

**FIGURE 2-38, cont'd D,** Same radiograph as **A** with structures labeled. Note irregular alveolar bone margins common in older animals and those that have had periodontitis.

1. First incisor tooth (*dentes incisivi*)
2. Second incisor tooth (*dentes incisivi*)
3. Third incisor tooth (*dentes incisivi*)
4. Canine tooth (*dentes canini*)
5. Alveolar bone margin, labial—apical to normal position due to pathology (*margo alveolaris*)
6. Alveolar bone margin, lingual—apical to normal position due to pathology (*margo alveolaris*)
7. Cervical burn-out caused by a relative lack of superimposed structures
8. Coronal enamel (accentuated due to tangential effect) (*enamelum*)
9. Dentin (*dentinum*)
10. Mandibular symphysis (*synchondrosis intermandibularis*)
11. Mental foramen—rostral (*foramen mentale*)
12. Periodontal ligament space (*periodontium, articulatio dentoalveolaris*)
13. Pulp chamber (*cavum coronale dentis, pulpa coronalis*)
14. Root canal space (*canalis radicis dentis, pulpa radicularis*)

## MANDIBULAR INCISOR TEETH

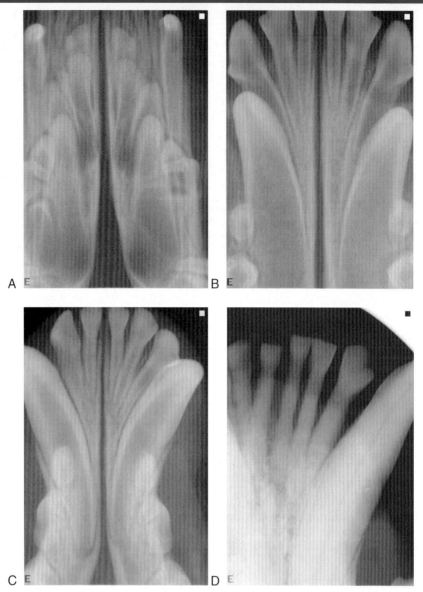

**FIGURE 2-39  Effect of age on incisor teeth.  A,** Three-month-old Standard Poodle. The apices are open with no constriction (see Chapter 2, Deciduous Teeth). **B,** Six-month-old Golden Retriever. The apices are still wide open but have some apical constriction. **C,** Eight-month-old Miniature Poodle. The apices have a pronounced constriction and the dentin walls are thicker. This dog is missing the right second incisor tooth. **D,** Five-year-old German Shepherd.

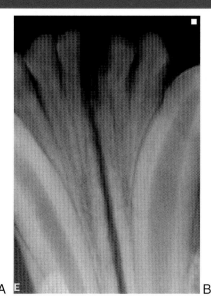 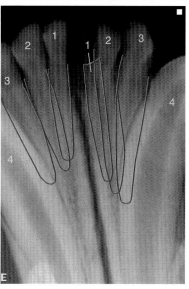

FIGURE 2-40 **A** and **B,** Apparent crowding of the incisor roots seen in two-dimensional radiographs seems to leave no room for periodontal supportive bone. The superimposed roots give the appearance of occupying the same space. Periodontal ligaments crossing roots can create radiolucent lines that mimic root fractures. **C** and **D,** Although the crowns of the incisor teeth normally sit side-by-side in the arch, in narrow-jawed dogs the relationship of the roots changes toward the apices as the second incisor roots are positioned dorsal to the roots of the first and third incisor teeth.

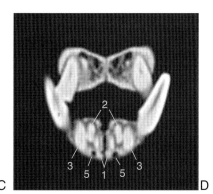 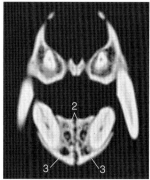

FIGURE 2-40, cont'd **C,** On a CT transverse plane image close to the apex of the first incisor root the second incisor root is positioned dorsal to the first and third. **D,** On a transverse plane image at the level of the apices of the second and third incisor roots, the second incisor root apex is positioned dorsal to the third incisor root apex.

1. First incisor tooth
2. Second incisor tooth
3. Third incisor tooth
4. canine tooth
5. nutrient canal

## MANDIBULAR CANINE TEETH

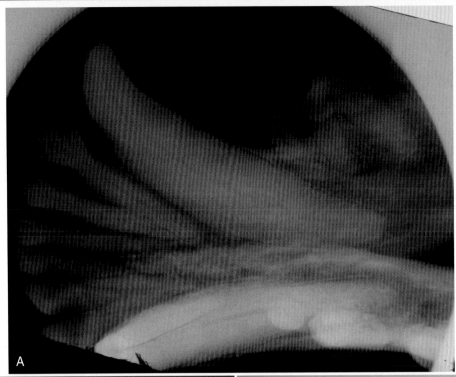

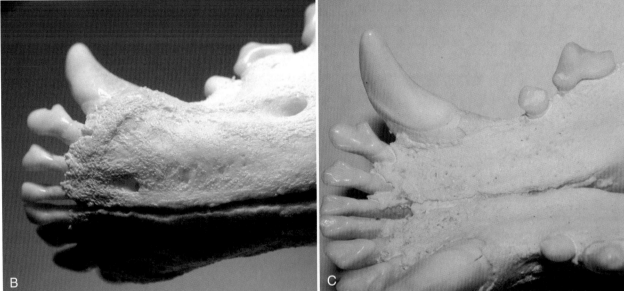

**FIGURE 2-41 Normal mandibular canine tooth. A,** Radiograph of the rostral mandibles from a mature dog includes the canine tooth and surrounding structures. The narrow pulp chamber and root canal spaces establish this to be from an older dog. **B,** Labial view of prepared mandibles. **C,** Lingual (mirror view) of the mandibles.

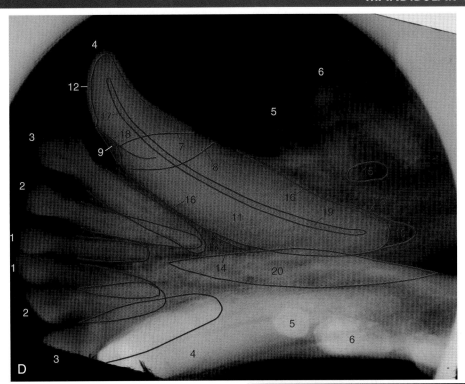

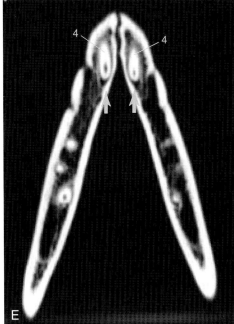

**FIGURE 2-41, cont'd D,** Same radiograph as **A. E,** a CT dorsal plane image of the mandibles at the level of the canine root tips. Hypoattenuation (*arrows*) around the apices is caused by the lack of apical bone that contributes to the radiographic chevron lucency.

1. First incisor tooth (*dentes incisivi*)
2. Second incisor tooth (*dentes incisivi*)
3. Third incisor tooth (*dentes incisivi*)
4. Canine tooth (*dentes canini*)
5. First premolar tooth (*dentes premolares*)
6. Second premolar tooth (*dentes premolares*)
7. Alveolar margin—labial (*margo alveolaris*)
8. Alveolar margin—lingual (*margo alveolaris*)
9. Cervical burnout
10. Chevron lucency
11. Dentin (*dentinum*)
12. Enamel (*enamelum*)
13. Lamina dura (*alveoli dentales*)
14. Mandibular symphysis (*synchondrosis intermandibularis*)
15. Middle mental foramen (*foramen mentale*)
16. Periodontal ligament space (*periodontium, articulatio dentoalveolaris*)
17. Pulp chamber (*cavum coronale dentis, pulpa coronalis*)
18. Ridge along the mesiolingual and lingual surfaces of the canine tooth.
19. Root canal (*canalis radicis dentis, pulpa radicularis*)
20. Superimposition of the right and left mandibles—lingual, ventral, and symphyseal surfaces

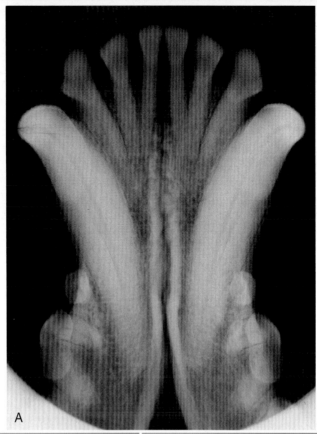

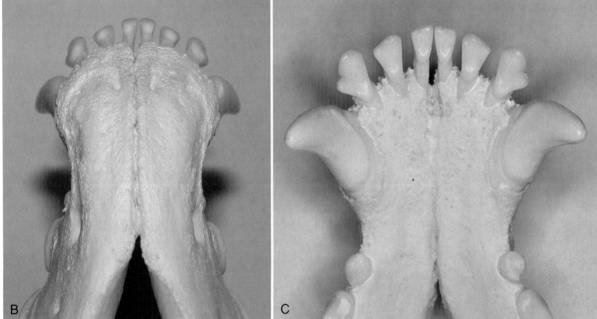

**FIGURE 2-42** A near-VD projection (see Chapter 12) displays both mandibular canine teeth side-by-side for comparison. **A,** Radiograph of the rostral mandibles from a mature dog showing the canine tooth and surrounding structures. **B,** Labial view of prepared mandibles. **C,** Lingual (mirror image) view of mandibles.

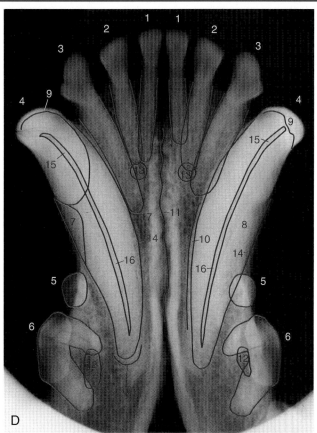

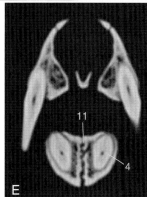

FIGURE 2-42, cont'd **D,** Same radiograph as **A. E,** On a CT transverse plane image, the symphysis is a joint and does not fuse even in an older animal. The symphyseal cortical bone plate of each mandible is oriented parallel to the x-ray beam on a ventrodorsal projection resulting in a very opaque line on a radiograph.

1. First incisor tooth (*dentes incisivi*)
2. Second incisor tooth (*dentes incisivi*)
3. Third incisor tooth (*dentes incisivi*)
4. Canine tooth (*dentes canini*)
5. First premolar tooth (*dentes premolares*)
6. Second premolar tooth (*dentes premolares*)
7. Cervical burnout
8. Dentin (*dentinum*)
9. Enamel (*enamelum*)
10. Lamina dura (*alveoli dentales*)
11. Mandibular symphysis (*synchondrosis intermandibularis*)
12. Mental foramen—middle (*foramen mentale*)
13. Mental foramen—rostral (*foramen mentale*)
14. Periodontal ligament space (*periodontium, articulatio dentoalveolaris*)
15. Pulp chamber (*cavum coronale dentis, pulpa coronalis*)
16. Root canal (*canalis radicis dentis, pulpa radicularis*)
17. Trabecular bone (*substantia spongiosa ossium*)

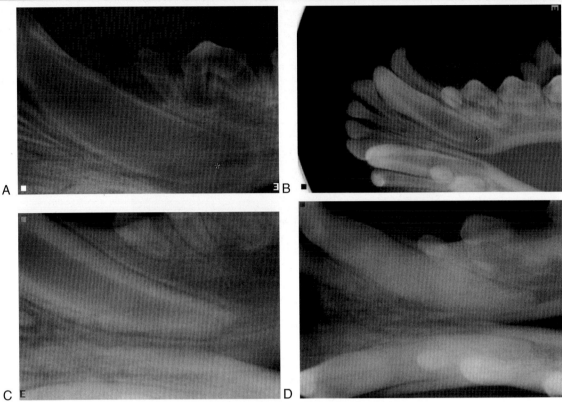

FIGURE 2-43 Effect of aging on the size of the pulp chambers and root canals of mandibular canine teeth in dogs. **A,** Four-month-old Belgian Malinois. The apex is wide open with no constriction (*asterisk*). **B,** Eight-month-old Yorkshire Terrier. The apices of the canine teeth are open (*asterisk*). This patient also has linguoversion of the mandibular canine teeth, two persistent deciduous canine teeth, and two missing incisor teeth. **C,** One-year-old Leonburger. The apex is closed but the pulp chamber is still quite large. **D,** Eight-year-old German Shepherd. The root canal is very narrow due to secondary dentin formation.

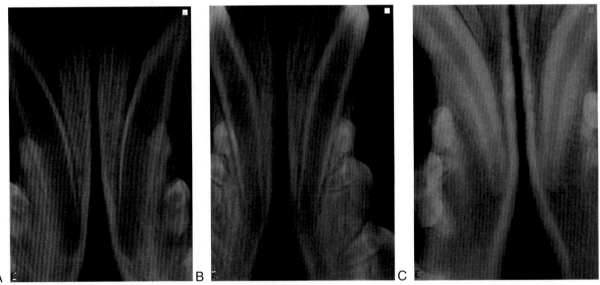

FIGURE 2-44 Ventrodorsal projection of mandibles from young dogs. **A,** Four-month-old Border Collie. Open apices with no constriction. **B,** Six-month-old Australian Shepherd. **C,** One-year-old Terrier. The root apices of the canine teeth are completely closed.

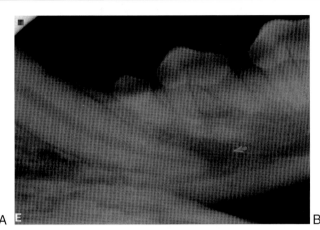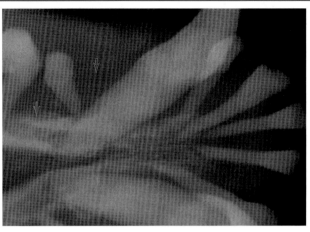

A  B

**FIGURE 2-45 Commonly found pathology. A,** Endodontic disease (see Chapter 6). Inflammation secondary to pulp inflammation or necrosis often causes periapical lucency (*arrow*). **B,** Periodontitis (see Chapter 5). Horizontal alveolar bone loss has decreased vertical dimension of the mandible, moving the alveolar margin apically (*arrow*) from its original position at the level of the *open arrow*.

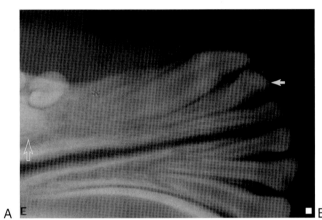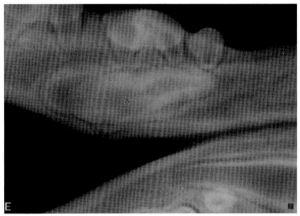

A  B

**FIGURE 2-46 Radiographs of the mandibles of a dog that was missing the right mandibular canine tooth. A,** The tooth is not present in its normal position (*asterisk*). Note also dilaceration of the right mandibular second incisor tooth (*arrow*) and rotation of the third incisor tooth. The tip of a radiopaque structure (*open arrow*) can be seen close to the left edge of the radiograph. **B,** This radiograph was made caudal to the one in **A.** The deformed and unerupted canine tooth is malpositioned caudally (asterisk) in the mandible. Trauma to a region of developing teeth in puppies can cause multiple teeth in one region to be affected by developmental abnormalities (see Chapters 9 and 10).

**MANDIBULAR PREMOLAR TEETH**

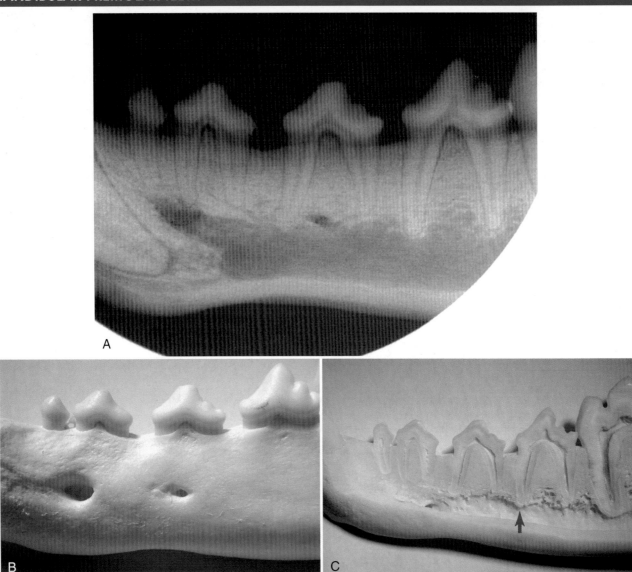

**FIGURE 2-47 Normal mandibular premolar teeth. A,** Radiograph of the left mandibular premolar teeth of a young dog. **B,** Buccal view of a prepared mandible. **C,** Buccal view of mandible that has had the buccal portion removed to view the relationship of the premolar teeth roots to the mandibular canal. Some premolar roots appear to protrude into the mandibular canal. The mesial root of the fourth premolar tooth (*arrow*) is positioned lingual to the canal but the apical alveolar bone protrudes slightly into the canal space.

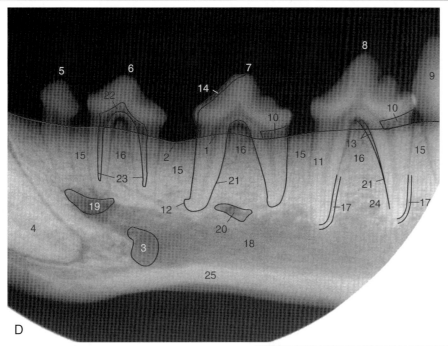

D

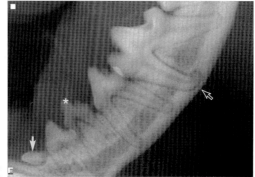

E

**FIGURE 2-47, cont'd D,** Same radiograph as **A. E,** Small breed dogs have a larger tooth-to-bone ratio. This results in the radiographic appearance of roots that pass completely through the mandibular canal. This patient also has an embedded first premolar tooth (*arrow*), a persistent deciduous third premolar tooth with no succedaneous permanent tooth (*asterisk*), and a dilacerated root tip of the mesial root of the first molar tooth (*open arrow*).

1. Alveolar margin (*margo alveolaris*)
2. Alveolar margin, interdental (*margo interalveolaris*)
3. Bifurcation of the mandibular canal into the most rostral section that travels lingual to the canine root
4. Canine tooth (*dentes canini*)
5. First premolar tooth (*dentes premolares*)
6. Second premolar tooth (*dentes premolares*)
7. Third premolar tooth (*dentes premolares*)
8. Fourth premolar tooth (*dentes premolares*)
9. First molar tooth (*dentes molares*)
10. Cervical burn-out caused by a relative lack of superimposed structures
11. Dentin (*dentinum*)
12. Dilacerated root tip
13. Double root shadow caused by radicular developmental groove
14. Enamel (*enamelum*)
15. Interalveolar septum (*septa interalveolaria*)
16. Interradicular bone (*septa interradicularia*)
17. Lamina dura (*alveoli dentales*)
18. Mandibular canal (*canalis mandibulae*)
19. Mental foramen, middle (*foramina mentalia*)
20. Mental foramen, caudal (*foramina mentalia*)
21. Periodontal ligament space (*periodontium, articulatio dentoalveolari*)
22. Pulp chamber (*cavum coronale dentis, pulpa coronalis*)
23. Root canal (*canalis radicis dentis, pulpa radicularis*)
24. Trabecular bone (*substantia spongiosa ossium*)
25. Ventral mandibular cortex (*margo ventralis*)

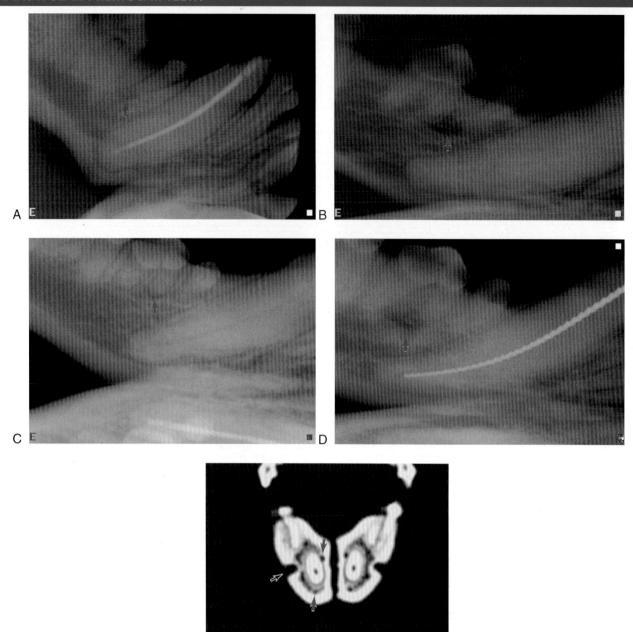

**FIGURE 2-48** The middle mental foramen most commonly exits ventral to the septal bone between the first and second premolar teeth, but the position can vary in some individuals. The radiographic lucency of the middle foramen (*arrows*) can be projected to **A,** the apex of the first premolar tooth; **B,** the area between the roots of the first and second premolar teeth; **C,** the apex of the mesial (rostral) root of the second premolar tooth; or **D,** the interradicular bone between the roots of the second premolar tooth. The lucency of the foramen can mimic a lesion of endodontic origin. **E,** CT scan transverse plane image at the level of the mesial root of the second premolar teeth. The foramen (*open arrow*) is further ventral to the premolar root tips than it appears on a radiograph, and it can be labial to the root of the canine tooth but is projected coronally on a dental radiograph. The CT image also shows multiple nutrient canals (*arrows*). The caudal mental foramen is usually positioned between the roots of the third premolar tooth but can also vary between individuals.

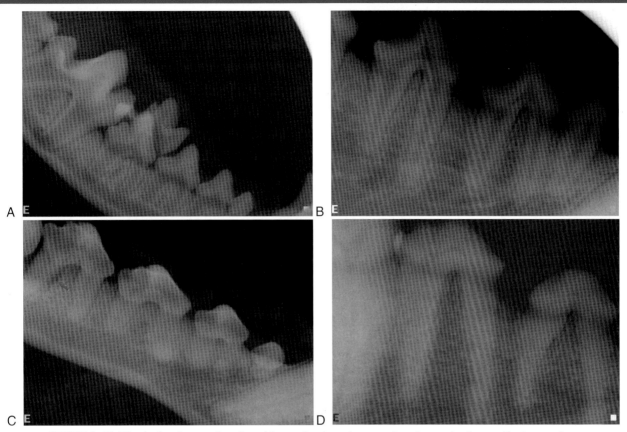

**FIGURE 2-49** Effect of aging on the size of the pulp chambers and root canals of mandibular canine teeth in dogs. **A,** Eight-month-old Yorkshire Terrier. The apices are open. The roots of the third deciduous premolar tooth have resorbed but the cap has not yet exfoliated (*asterisk*). **B,** One-year-old Yellow Labrador. The apices have closed and the dentin walls are thicker. **C,** Five-year-old Miniature Schnauzer. The pulp cavities are much smaller. The distal root of the fourth premolar has vertical bone loss (*arrow*). **D,** Eleven-year-old Golden Retriever. The pulp chambers and root canal spaces are even smaller. The cusp tips are flattened from abrasional wear.

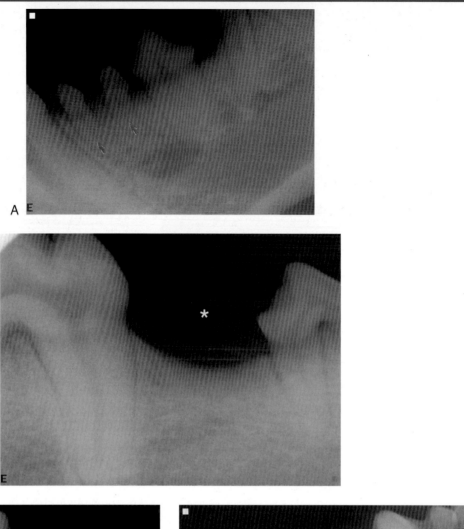

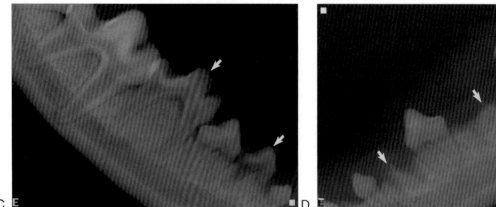

**FIGURE 2-50** Congenital polyodontia and hypodontia (see Chapter 9). **A,** Supernumerary first premolar tooth (*arrows*). **B,** The right mandibular fourth premolar tooth is missing (*asterisk*). Absence of permanent premolar teeth is a common finding in some breeds of dog. **C,** The right mandible has persistent deciduous second and fourth premolar teeth occupying the spaces with no underlying permanent teeth (*arrows*). The deciduous second premolar tooth has a large radiolucent area in the distal root indicating that resorption is occurring and the tooth will likely exfoliate. **D,** The left mandible from the same dog and at the same time as the radiograph in **C.** The deciduous second and fourth premolar teeth have already exfoliated, and there are no succedaneous permanent teeth to replace them (*arrows*).

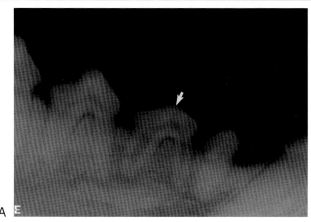
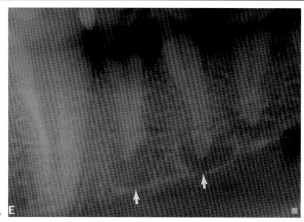

A

B

**FIGURE 2-51 Endodontic disease (see Chapter 6). A,** The right mandibular second premolar tooth has a wider pulp cavity than the adjacent teeth (*arrow*). This is consistent with a necrotic pulp that stopped maturing while the adjacent healthy teeth continued to produce secondary dentin. **B,** The right mandibular fourth premolar tooth has periapical lucencies with radiopaque borders (*arrows*), indicating chronic lesions of endodontic origin.

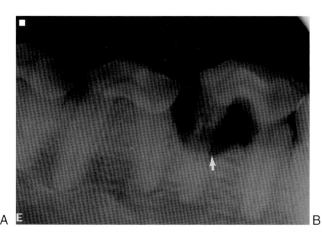
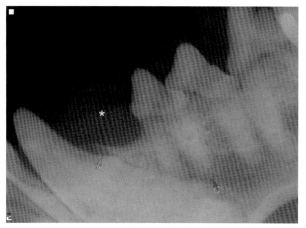

A

B

**FIGURE 2-52 Miscellaneous findings. A,** Periodontitis (see Chapter 5). Oblique and horizontal alveolar bone loss affects the mesial root of the left mandibular fourth premolar tooth (*arrow*). **B,** Multiple findings on a 9-year-old Lhasa Apso. The distal root of the second premolar tooth is superimposed over the mesial root of the third premolar (*arrow*) due to rotation and crowding. The first premolar tooth is missing (*asterisk*). The canine tooth is incompletely erupted with a resultant pseudopocket due to the sulcular enamel (*open arrow*).

## MANDIBULAR MOLAR TEETH

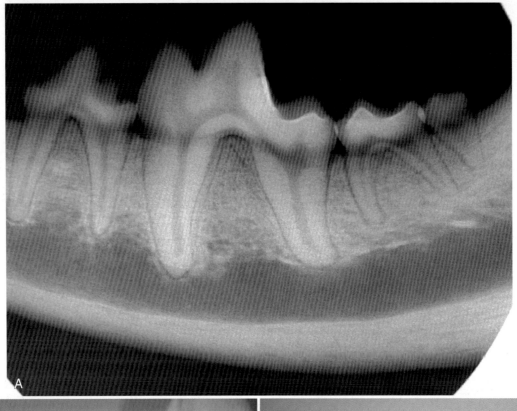

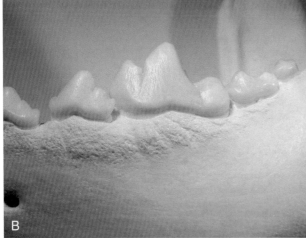

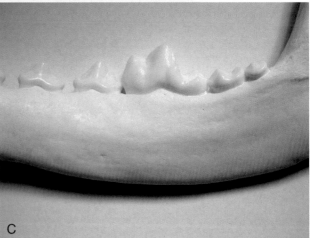

FIGURE 2-53 **Normal mandibular molar teeth. A,** Radiograph of the left mandibular molar teeth of a young dog. **B,** Buccal view of prepared mandible. **C,** Lingual (mirror image) view. **D** (*facing page top*), Same radiograph as **A. E,** Buccal view of mandible that has had bone removed to uncover the mandibular canal. **F,** Buccal view with additional bone removed to the level of the lingual wall of the mandibular canal. The relationship of the molar tooth roots to the canal lumen is visible. In this relatively large dog, the distal (caudal) root of the mandibular first molar tooth is dorsal to the canal roof. The apical extent of the cortical alveolar bone of the mesial (rostral) root protrudes into the lumen of the canal but is located mostly dorsolingual to the canal.

1. Alveolar margin (*margo alveolaris*)
2. Cervical burn-out
3. Dentin (*dentinum*)
4. Enamel (*enamelum*)
5. Interalveolar margin (*margo interalveolaris*)
6. Interdental alveolar septum (*septa interalveolaria*)
7. Interradicular bone (*septa interradicularia*)

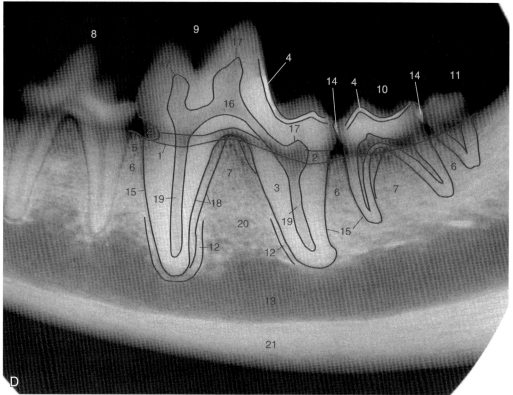

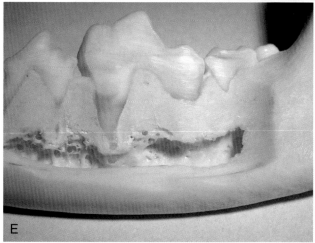

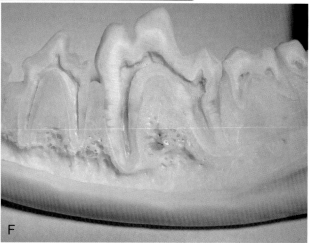

8. Fourth premolar tooth (*dentes premolares*)
9. First molar tooth (*dentes molares*)
10. Second molar tooth (*dentes molares*)
11. Third molar tooth (*dentes molares*)
12. Lamina dura—compact bone of alveolar wall (*alveoli dentales*)
13. Mandibular canal (*canalis mandibulae*)
14. Overlap of proximal enamel (summation)
15. Periodontal ligament space (*periodontium, articulatio dentoalveolaris*)
16. Pulp chamber (*cavum coronale dentis, pulpa coronalis*)
17. Pulp horn
18. Radicular groove
19. Root canal (*canalis radicis dentis, pulpa radicularis*)
20. Trabecular bone (*substantia spongiosa ossium*)
21. Ventral mandibular cortex (*margo ventralis*)

**MANDIBULAR MOLAR TEETH**

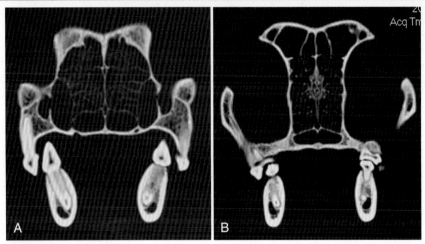

**FIGURE 2-54 CT scan transverse plane images.** The root tips of the first molar tooth are dorsal and lingual to the mandibular canal in this medium-sized dog. **A,** At the level of the mesial (rostral) root. **B,** At the level of the distal (caudal) root.

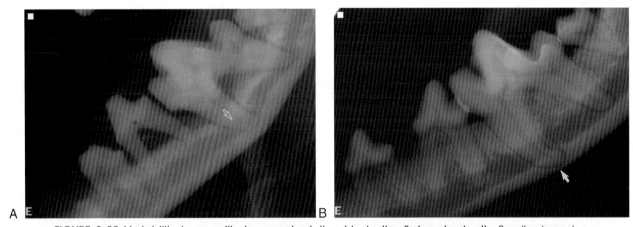

**FIGURE 2-55 Variability in mandibular canal relationship to the first molar tooth.** Smaller breeds have a larger tooth-to-bone ratio than larger breeds. **A,** In this dog, the mandibular canal appears to deviate ventrally as it crosses the molar roots (*open arrow*). This dog also has alveolar bone loss from periodontitis, super-eruption of the fourth premolar tooth (*asterisk*), a cusp tip fracture of the third premolar tooth, and a missing second premolar tooth with a persistent distal root fragment. **B,** In very small breeds, the apex of the mesial (rostral) root of the mandibular first molar tooth can be very close to the ventral mandibular cortex (*arrow*).

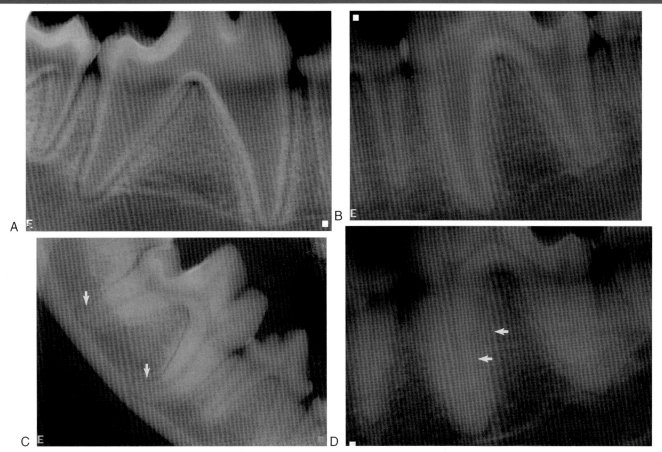

**FIGURE 2-56** Effect of aging on the size of the pulp chambers and root canals of mandibular first molar teeth in dogs. **A,** Six-month-old Golden Retriever. The apices are nearly closed and the dentin walls are quite thin. **B,** One-year-old Labrador Retriever. The apices are completely closed and more dentin has been deposited on the periphery of the pulp cavity. **C,** Two-year-old Toy Poodle. The dentin walls are thicker due to secondary dentin deposition. The apical sections of both roots are dilacerated with distinct distal angulation (*arrows*). This is the result of continued root development after complete eruption in a small-breed dog with a high tooth-to-bone ratio. **D,** Nine-year-old Dalmation mix. There is marked attenuation of the pulp chamber and root canal spaces. This molar tooth has a very distinct double-shadow due to a deep radicular groove on the distal aspect of the mesial root (*arrows*).

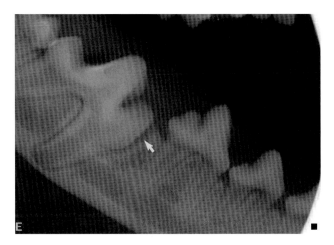

**FIGURE 2-57** Poorly erupted mandibular first molar tooth in a Maltese (see Chapter 9). There is a pseudopocket adjacent to the unerupted portion of the mesial crown (*arrow*). The pseudopocket occurs because periodontal tissues cannot form an attachment to enamel.

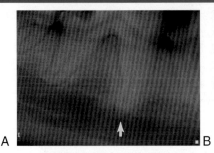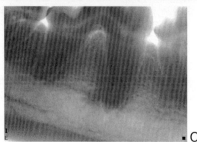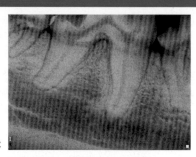

A     B     C

**FIGURE 2-58** Summation of the mandibular canal superimposed over the apices of the first molar tooth can mimic an endodontic lesion. **A,** Radiograph of a right mandibular first molar tooth with a radiolucency at the apex of the mesial root where it is superimposed over the canal (*arrow*). The lamina dura is lost at the root tip. **B,** A reverse (negative) image helps to visualize the intact periodontal ligament space (white line in the reverse image) that remains intact around the root tip. **C,** An enhanced image ("revealer mode"; see Chapter 13) increases the contrast to facilitate visualization of the intact periodontal ligament space around the root tip. The root tip does have an irregular shape indicating possible external resorption. The significance of this is unclear; follow-up radiographs are needed to look for changes.

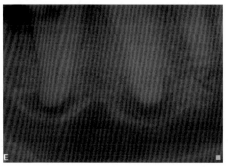

**FIGURE 2-59** Endodontic disease (see Chapter 6). A periapical endodontic lesion can have its own expanded radiopaque lamina dura in chronic cases. In this radiograph the normal lamina dura of the alveolus is lost, and the periapical periodontal ligament space is gone.

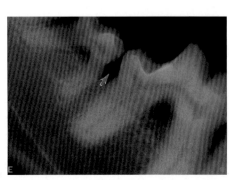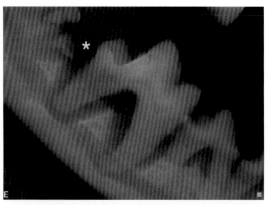

A     B

**FIGURE 2-60** Periodontal disease (see Chapter 5). **A,** There is bone loss in the furcation area of the molar tooth and in the interproximal area between the molar teeth (*arrow*). **B,** Infection has caused bone loss and resulted in secondary endodontic disease. The mesial crown-root segment of the second molar tooth is missing (*asterisk*). Periodontitis affects the premolar teeth and all three molar teeth in this patient.

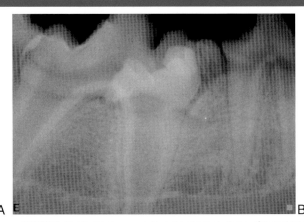
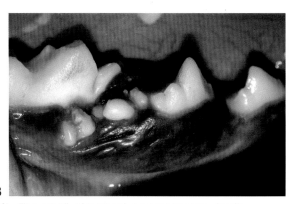

**FIGURE 2-61 Compound odontoma (see Chapter 8).** The small abnormal supernumerary teeth associated with the mandibular molar are typical of a compound odontoma.

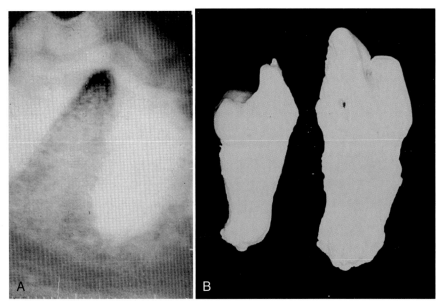

**FIGURE 2-62 Ankylosis in a geriatric dog. A,** Radiograph shows generalized loss of the periodontal ligament space and lamina dura along the entire root outline. **B,** The extracted tooth demonstrates the very rough and thickened root surface.

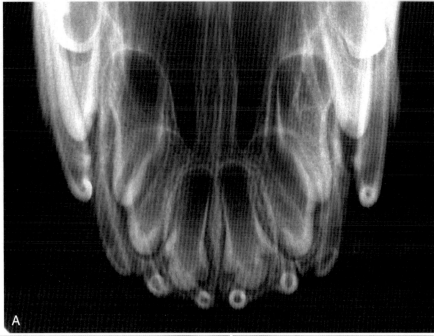

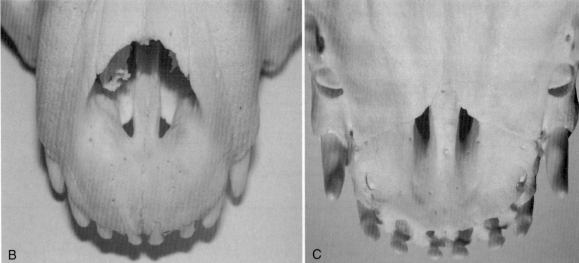

FIGURE 2-63 Normal maxillary deciduous incisor teeth. **A,** Radiograph of the incisor teeth and rostral maxillary region of a puppy with a deciduous dentition. **B,** Dorsal view of prepared skull. **C,** Ventral (mirror image) view of skull.

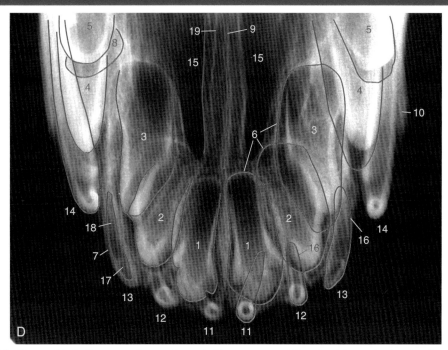

**FIGURE 2-63, cont'd D,** Same radiograph as **A.** The crowns of the deciduous incisor teeth are fore-shortened due to a near-parallel orientation to the x-ray beam because of their curvature. The roots of the deciduous incisors are positioned labial to the developing permanent teeth. The deciduous tooth roots are in the eruption pathway of the permanent teeth. The presence, proximity, and correct location of the developing permanent teeth all play an important role in the process of deciduous tooth exfoliation. The permanent incisor tooth buds already have radiographically recognizable pulp, dentin, and enamel components.

1. Permanent first incisor tooth (*dentes permanentes, dentes incisivi*)
2. Permanent second incisor tooth (*dentes permanentes, dentes incisivi*)
3. Permanent third incisor tooth (*dentes permanentes, dentes incisivi*)
4. Permanent canine tooth (*dentes permanentes, dentes canini*)
5. Permanent first premolar tooth (*dentes permanentes, dentes premolares*)
6. Bony crypt of permanent tooth follicle
7. Dentin (*dentinum*)
8. Gubernacular foramen
9. Interincisive suture (*sutura interincisiva*)
10. Maxilla (*corpus maxillae*)
11. Deciduous first incisor tooth (*dentes decidui, dentes incisivi*)
12. Deciduous second incisor tooth (*dentes decidui, dentes incisivi*)
13. Deciduous third incisor tooth (*dentes decidui, dentes incisivi*)
14. Deciduous canine tooth (*dentes decidui, dentes canini*)
15. Palatine fissure (*fissura palatina*)
16. Periodontal ligament space (*periodontium, articulatio dentoalveolari*)
17. Pulp chamber (*cavum coronale dentis, pulpa coronalis*)
18. Root canal (*canalis radicis dentis, pulpa radicularis*)
19. Vomer

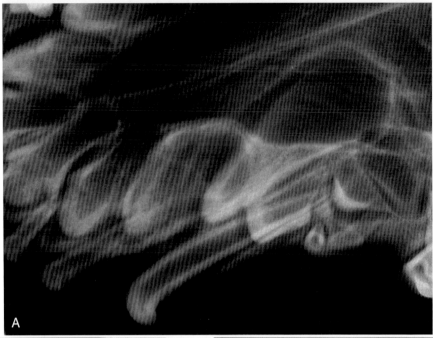

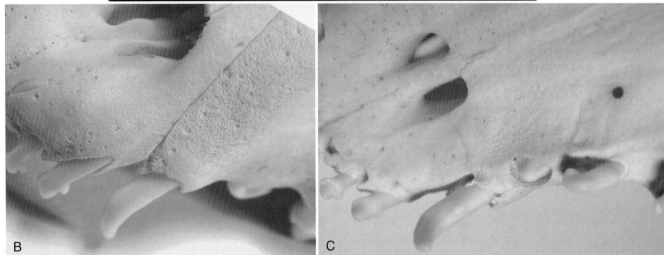

**FIGURE 2-64 Normal deciduous canine tooth. A,** Radiograph of the canine tooth and surrounding structures of a puppy in the deciduous dentition stage. **B,** Labial view of prepared skull. **C,** Palatal (mirror image) view of skull.

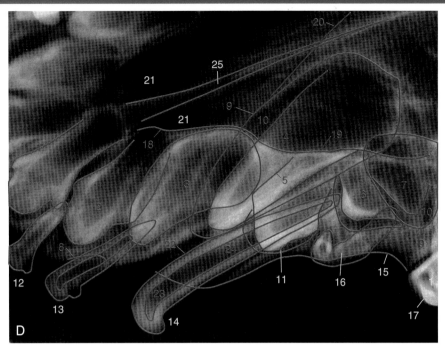

**FIGURE 2-64, cont'd  D,** Same radiograph as **A.** The underlying succedaneous permanent teeth are superimposed over the deciduous teeth. The palatal surface of the incisive bone and maxilla have open foramena at future eruption sites even though the soft tissues show no evidence of the erupting permanent teeth at this age. The majority of the radiolucency coronal to the developing crowns is a result of the eruption cyst; a normal part of the eruption process.

1. Permanent first incisor tooth (*dentes permanentes, dentes incisivi*)
2. Permanent second incisor tooth (*dentes permanentes, dentes incisivi*)
3. Permanent third incisor tooth (*dentes permanentes, dentes incisivi*)
4. Permanent canine tooth (*dentes permanentes, dentes canini*)
5. Permanent first premolar tooth (*dentes permanentes, dentes premolares*)
6. Permanent second premolar tooth (*dentes permanentes, dentes premolares*)
7. Permanent third premolar tooth (*dentes permanentes, dentes premolares*)
8. Alveolar margin—buccal (*margo alveolaris*)
9. Bony crypt of permanent tooth follicle
10. Eruption cyst
11. Gubernacular foramen
12. Deciduous second incisor tooth (*dentes decidui, dentes incisivi*)
13. Deciduous third incisor tooth (*dentes decidui, dentes incisivi*)
14. Deciduous canine tooth (*dentes decidui, dentes canini*)
15. Interdental alveolar margin—palatal (*margo interalveolaris*)
16. Deciduous second premolar tooth (*dentes decidui, dentes premolares*)
17. Deciduous third premolar tooth (*dentes decidui, dentes premolares*)
18. Nasal surface of the alveolar process of incisive bone (*os incisivum, processus alveolaris*)
19. Nasal surface of alveolar process of the maxilla (*facies nasalis, processus alveolaris*)
20. Incisivomaxillary suture (*sutura incisivomaxillaris*)
21. Palatine fissure (*fissura palatina*)
22. Periodontal ligament space (*periodontium, articulatio dentoalveolari*)
23. Pulp chamber (*cavum coronale dentis, pulpa coronalis*)
24. Root canal (*canalis radicis dentis, pulpa radicularis*)
25. Vomer

## DECIDUOUS TEETH

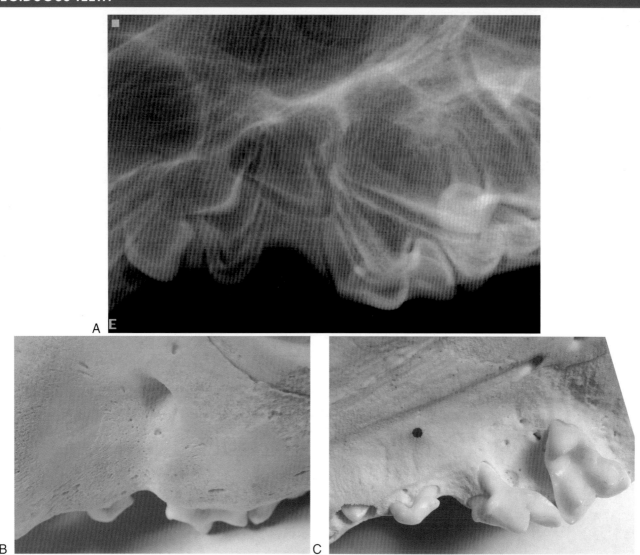

**FIGURE 2-65 Normal maxillary deciduous premolar teeth. A,** Radiograph of the premolar teeth and surrounding structures of a puppy in the deciduous dentition stage. **B,** Buccal view of prepared skull. **C,** Palatal (mirror image) view of skull.

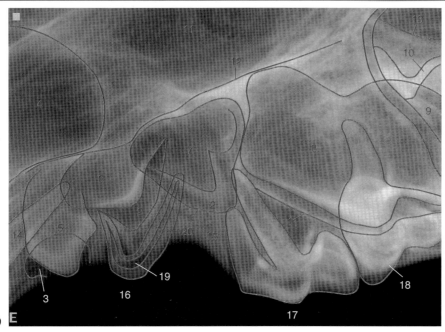

**FIGURE 2-65, cont'd  D,** Same radiograph as **A.** Dogs have only three deciduous premolar teeth and no deciduous molar teeth. The deciduous teeth function as a temporary dentition for a puppy's small jaws. As the jaws get larger and more powerful, the permanent dentition replaces the deciduous teeth with the more numerous and larger teeth required for an adult. The deciduous premolar teeth are the second, third, and fourth premolars due to their relationship with their successors rather than due to their function or anatomy.

1. Bony crypt of permanent tooth follicle
2. Eruption cyst
3. Gubernacular foramen
4. Permanent canine tooth (*dentes permanentes, dentes canini*)
5. Permanent first premolar tooth (*dentes permanentes, dentes premolares*)
6. Permanent second premolar tooth (*dentes permanentes, dentes premolares*)
7. Permanent third premolar tooth (*dentes permanentes, dentes premolares*)
8. Permanent fourth premolar tooth (*dentes permanentes, dentes premolares*)
9. First molar tooth (*dentes molares*)
10. First molar tooth—enamel of developing palatal cusp
11. Nasal cavity (*cavum nasi*)
12. Nasal surface of alveolar process of the maxilla (*facies nasalis, processus alveolaris*)
13. Orbital rim (*os zygomaticum, margo infraorbitalis*)
14. Deciduous canine tooth (*dentes decidui, dentes canini*)
15. Periodontal ligament space (*periodontium, articulatio dentoalveolari*)
16. Deciduous second premolar tooth (*dentes decidui, dentes premolares*)
17. Deciduous third premolar tooth (*dentes decidui, dentes premolares*)
18. Deciduous fourth premolar tooth (*dentes decidui, dentes premolares*
19. Pulp chamber (*cavum coronale dentis, pulpa coronalis*)
20. Root canal (*canalis radicis dentis, pulpa radicularis*)

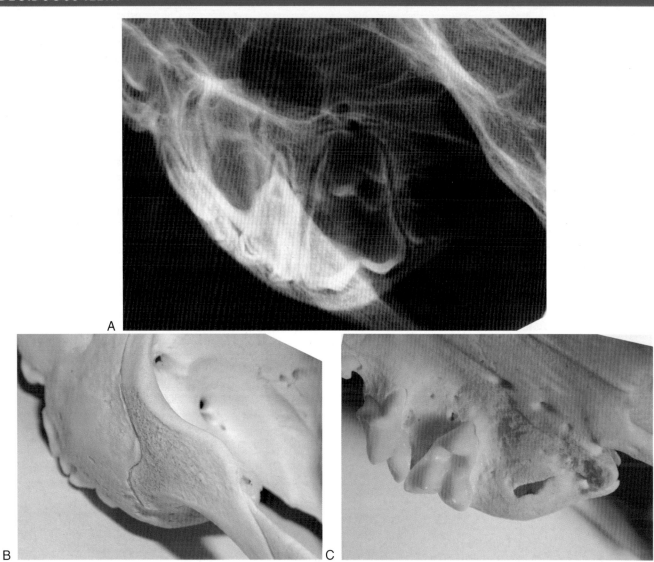

A

B                                                                C

**FIGURE 2-66 Developing permanent molar teeth. A,** Radiograph of the molar area of a puppy skull in the deciduous dentition stage. **B,** Buccal view of prepared skull. **C,** Palatal (mirror image) view of skull.

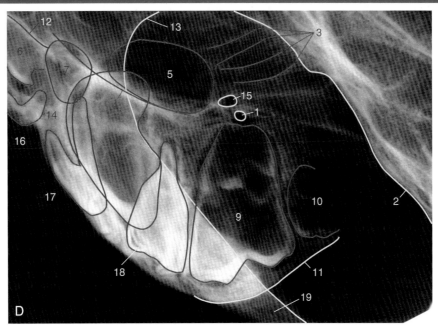

**FIGURE 2-66, cont'd  D,** Same radiograph as **A.** The molar area of the maxillary arch is edentulous in the deciduous dentition.

1. Caudal palatine foramen (*foramen palatinum caudale*)
2. Cranium—frontal, basisphenoid, and parietal bones (*cavum cranii—os frontale, os basisphenoidale, os parietale*)
3. Ethmoidal labyrinth (*labyrinthus ethmoidalis*)
4. Infraorbital canal wall (*canalis infraorbitalis*)
5. Maxillary recess (*recessus maxillaris*)
6. Permanent second premolar tooth (*dentes permanentes, dentes premolares*)
7. Permanent third premolar tooth (*dentes permanentes, dentes premolares*)
8. Permanent fourth premolar tooth (*dentes permanentes, dentes premolares*)
9. First molar tooth (*dentes molares*)
10. Second molar tooth (*dentes molares*)
11. Maxillary tuberosity (*tuber maxillae*)
12. Nasal surface of the alveolar process of the maxilla (*processus alveolaris*)
13. Orbital rim (*os zygomaticum, margo infraorbitalis*)
14. Periodontal ligament space (*periodontium, articulatio dentoalveolari*)
15. Sphenopalatine foramen (*foramen sphenopalatinum*)
16. Deciduous second premolar tooth (*dentes decidui, dentes premolares*)
17. Deciduous third premolar tooth (*dentes decidui, dentes premolares*)
18. Deciduous fourth premolar tooth (*dentes decidui, dentes premolares*)
19. Zygomatic bone (*os zygomaticum, processus temporalis*)

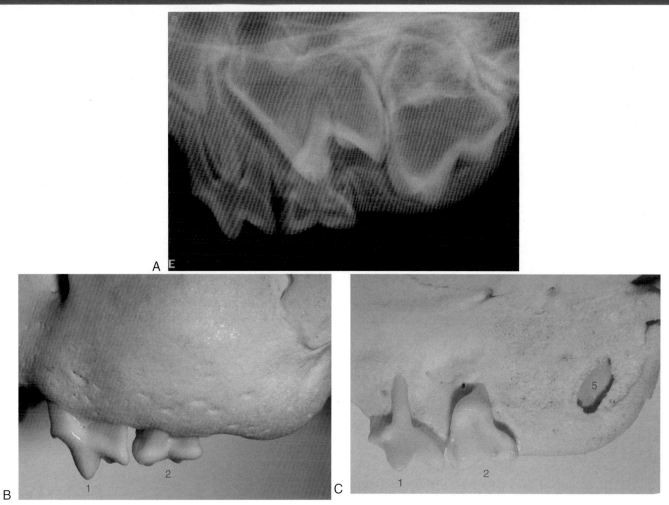

**FIGURE 2-67**  Third and fourth deciduous premolar anatomy and relationship to developing permanent premolars. **A,** Radiograph of the molar area of a puppy in the deciduous dentition stage. **B,** Buccal view of prepared skull. **C,** Palatal (mirror image) view of skull.

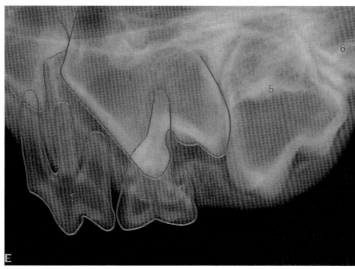

D E

**FIGURE 2-67, cont'd  D,** same radiograph as **A.** The anatomy of the deciduous third premolar tooth is similar to that of a permanent fourth premolar tooth with three roots and a carnassial crown. The anatomy of the deciduous fourth premolar tooth is similar to that of the permanent first molar tooth with a large occlusal surface.

1. Deciduous third premolar tooth
2. Deciduous fourth premolar tooth
3. Permanent third premolar tooth
4. Permanent fourth premolar tooth
5. First molar tooth
6. Second molar tooth

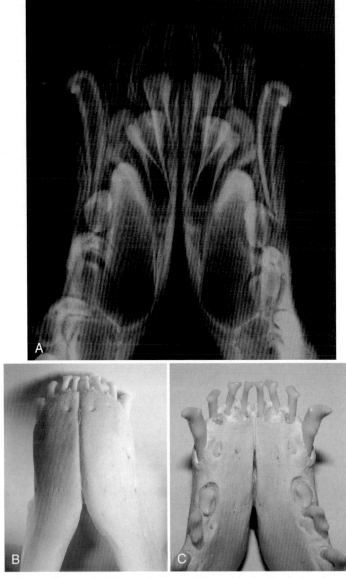

**FIGURE 2-68** Normal mandibular deciduous incisor and canine teeth. **A,** Radiograph of the incisor teeth and rostral mandibles of a puppy with a deciduous dentition. **B,** Ventral view of prepared mandibles. **C,** Dorsal (mirror image) view of mandibles.

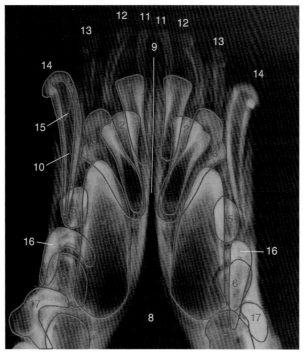

**FIGURE 2-68, cont'd D,** Same radiograph as **A.** The roots of the deciduous incisors are positioned labial to the developing permanent teeth.

1. Permanent first incisor tooth (*dentes permanentes, dentes incisivi*)
2. Permanent second incisor tooth (*dentes permanentes, dentes incisivi*)
3. Permanent third incisor tooth (*dentes permanentes, dentes incisivi*)
4. Permanent canine tooth (*dentes permanentes, dentes canini*)
5. Permanent first premolar tooth (*dentes permanentes, dentes premolares*)
6. Permanent second premolar tooth (*dentes permanentes, dentes premolares*)
7. Permanent third premolar tooth (*dentes permanentes, dentes premolares*)
8. Intermandibular space
9. Mandibular symphysis (*synchondrosis intermandibularis*)
10. Root canal (*canalis radicis dentis, pulpa radicularis*)
11. Deciduous first incisor tooth (*dentes decidui, dentes incisivi*)
12. Deciduous second incisor tooth (*dentes decidui, dentes incisivi*)
13. Deciduous third incisor tooth (*dentes decidui, dentes incisivi*)
14. Deciduous canine tooth (*dentes decidui, dentes canini*)
15. Ridge on lingual aspect of crown
16. Second deciduous premolar tooth—first is absent (*dentes decidui, dentes premolares*)
17. Third deciduous premolar tooth (*dentes decidui, dentes premolares*)

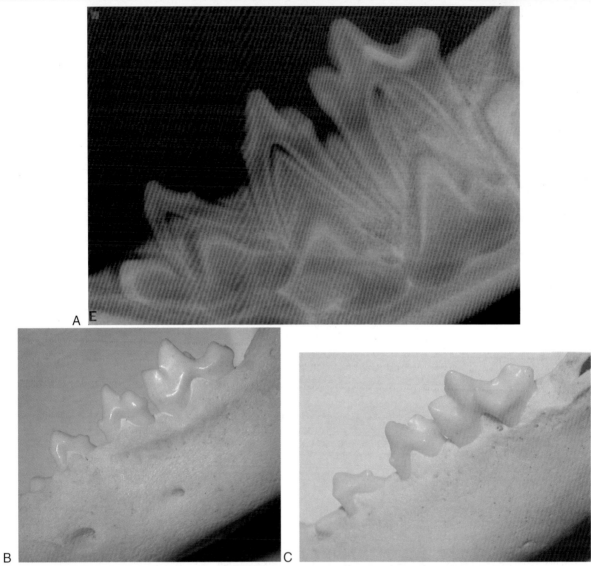

A

B

C

FIGURE 2-69 **Normal mandibular deciduous premolar teeth. A,** Radiograph of the premolar teeth and surrounding structures of a puppy in the deciduous dentition stage. **B,** Buccal view of prepared skull. **C,** palatal (mirror image) view of skull.

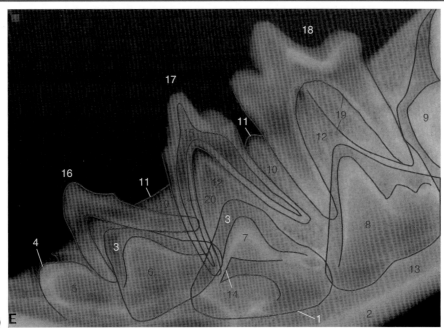

**FIGURE 2-69, cont'd D,** Same radiograph as **A.** Just as in the upper jaw, dogs have only three deciduous premolar teeth and no deciduous molar teeth. The deciduous premolar teeth are considered to be the second, third, and fourth premolars due to the teeth that succeed them in the jaw rather than due to their function or anatomy. The fourth deciduous premolar tooth has the morphology and function of a molar tooth, but is replaced by the permanent fourth premolar tooth.

1. Bony crypt of permanent tooth follicle
2. Compact bone of ventral mandible (*margo ventralis*)
3. Eruption cyst
4. Gubernacular foramen
5. Permanent first premolar tooth (*dentes permanentes, dentes premolares*)
6. Permanent second premolar tooth (*dentes permanentes, dentes premolares*)
7. Permanent third premolar tooth (*dentes permanentes, dentes premolares*)
8. Permanent fourth premolar tooth (*dentes permanentes, dentes premolares*)
9. First molar tooth (*dentes molares*)
10. Interalveolar septum (*septa interalveolaria*)
11. Interdental alveolar margin (*margo interalveolaris*)
12. Interradicular alveolar septum (*septa interradicularia*)
13. Mandibular canal (*canalis mandibulae*)
14. Mental foramen, caudal (*foramina mentalia*)
15. Pulp chamber (*cavum coronale dentis, pulpa coronalis*)
16. Deciduous second premolar tooth—dogs do not have a first deciduous premolar tooth (*dentes decidui, dentes premolares*)
17. Deciduous third premolar tooth (*dentes decidui, dentes premolares*)
18. Deciduous fourth premolar tooth (*dentes decidui, dentes premolares*)
19. Radicular groove—double periodontal ligament lucency
20. Root canal (*canalis radicis dentis, pulpa radicularis*)

# DECIDUOUS TEETH

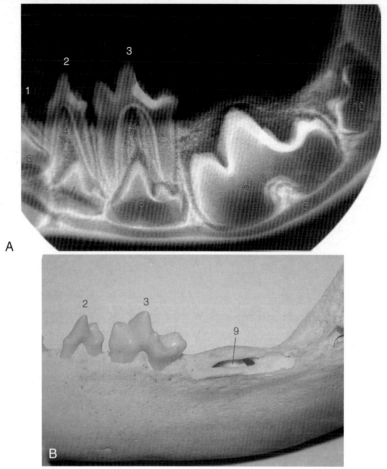

**FIGURE 2-70** Area of the developing molar teeth of the mandible from a puppy in the deciduous dentition period. **A,** Radiograph of the developing molar teeth. **B,** Picture of the lingual surface of a prepared mandible. The mandibular first molar tooth has a large gubernacular foramen. The molar area remains edentulous in the puppy until the permanent teeth erupt. The most commonly absent permanent molar tooth in the dog is the mandibular third molar. Missing this tooth may be considered a variation of normal in many small breeds of dogs.

1. Deciduous second premolar tooth—dogs do not have a first deciduous premolar tooth (*dentes decidui, dentes premolares*)
2. Deciduous third premolar tooth (*dentes decidui, dentes premolares*)
3. Deciduous fourth premolar tooth (*dentes decidui, dentes premolares*)
4. Interradicular alveolar septum (*septa interradicularia*)
5. Mandibular canal (*canalis mandibulae*)
6. Permanent second premolar tooth (*dentes permanentes, dentes premolares*)
7. Permanent third premolar tooth (*dentes permanentes, dentes premolares*)
8. Permanent fourth premolar tooth (*dentes permanentes, dentes premolares*)
9. First molar tooth (*dentes molares*)
10. Second molar tooth (*dentes molares*)

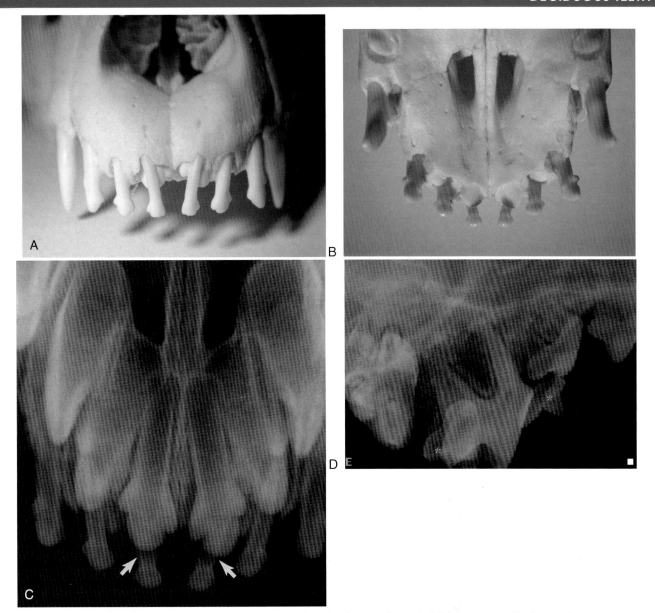

**FIGURE 2-71 Exfoliation of deciduous teeth. A,** Labial view of the skull from a puppy that was close to eruption of the maxillary first incisor teeth. **B,** Palatal view of the same skull preparation showing the permanent tooth crowns making direct contact with the deciduous teeth and erupting at an angle that would apply pressure to the roots. **C,** On a radiograph of the skull in **A** and **B,** the roots of the right and left first deciduous incisor teeth show resorption where the crowns of the permanent teeth are preparing to break through the gingiva (*arrows*). **D,** Radiograph of a dog in the mixed dentition period. There is root resorption of the deciduous third and fourth premolar teeth (*asterisks*) where the permanent teeth are erupting into their positions.

**DECIDUOUS TEETH**

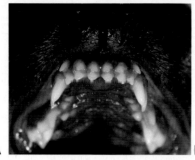
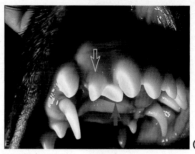
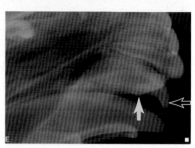

**FIGURE 2-72 Persistent deciduous teeth. A,** This Chihuahua failed to exfoliate the entire set of deciduous incisor teeth (labial set) because the permanent teeth erupted in the wrong position or angle to contribute to deciduous root resorption. **B,** This dog has a rotated and malpositioned right maxillary third permanent incisor tooth (*arrow*) and a persistent third deciduous incisor tooth (*open arrow*) occupying the space where the permanent tooth should be positioned. **C,** Radiograph of the dog in **B**.

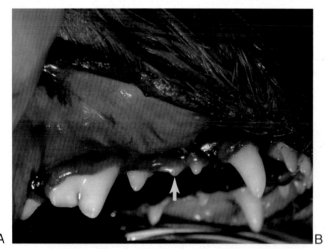
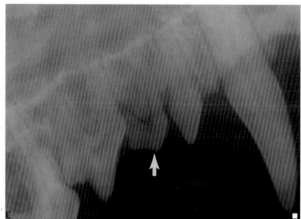

**FIGURE 2-73 Persistent deciduous premolar with no succedaneous permanent tooth. A,** The second premolar tooth is abnormally small (*arrow*). A tooth with an unusually small clinical crown is most commonly either a persistent deciduous tooth or an anomalous abnormally developed tooth. **B,** The radiograph confirms that the tooth is a deciduous tooth that has no underlying permanent tooth.

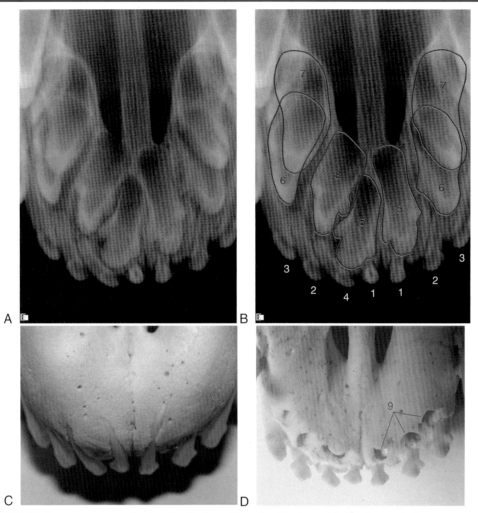

**FIGURE 2-74 Supernumerary incisor tooth (see Chapter 9). A** and **B,** Radiograph from a puppy in the deciduous dentition period. **C,** Labial view of skull prep from the same specimen as radiographed in **A. D,** Palatal view (mirror image) of the specimen. A supernumerary deciduous tooth may, but does not always, have a succedaneous supernumerary permanent tooth.

1. First deciduous incisor tooth
2. Second deciduous incisor tooth
3. Third deciduous incisor tooth
4. Supernumerary deciduous incisor tooth
5. First permanent incisor tooth
6. Second permanent incisor tooth
7. Third permanent incisor tooth
8. Supernumerary permanent incisor tooth
9. Gubernacular foramina

## SUGGESTED READINGS

Crossley DA: Tooth enamel thickness in the mature dentition of domestic dogs and cats – preliminary study, *J Vet Dent,* 12:111-113, 1995.

Gioso MA, Shofer F, Barros PFM, Harvey CE: Mandible and mandibular first molar tooth measurements in dogs: Relationship of radiographic height to body weight, *J Vet Dent,* 18:65–68, 2001.

Gorrel C: Radiographic evaluation: In: Holmstrom SE, editor: Canine dentistry, *Vet Clin N Am Small Anim Pract,* 28: 1089-1110, 1998.

International Committee on Veterinary Gross Anatomical Nomenclature: *Nomina anatomica veterinaria,* International Committee on Veterinary Gross Anatomical Nomenclature Editorial Committee, 2005. Available from www.wava-amav.org..

Miller ME, Christensen GC, Evans HE: *Anatomy of the dog,* Philadelphia, 1964, WB Saunders.

Schebitz H., Wilkens H: *Atlas of radiographic anatomy of the dog and cat,* ed 3, Philadelphia, 1978, Verlag Paul Parey/WB Saunders.

Wiggs RB, Lobprise HB: *Veterinary dentistry principles and practice,* Philadelphia, 1997, Lippincott-Raven.

# Intraoral Radiographic Anatomy of the Cat

## MAXILLARY INCISOR TEETH

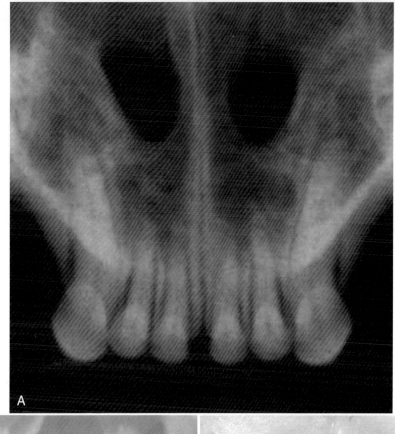

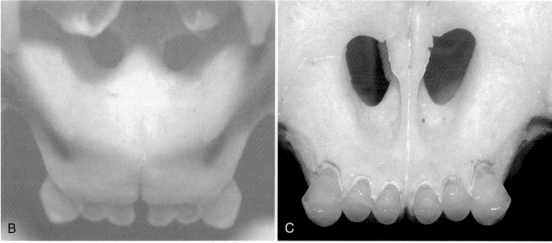

FIGURE 3-1 Normal incisor teeth in adult cat. **A,** Radiograph of the incisor teeth and rostral maxillary region of an adult cat skull. **B,** Dorsal view of prepared skull. **C,** Ventral (mirror) view of skull.

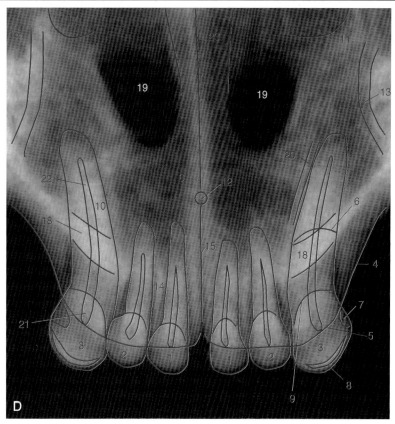

**FIGURE 3-1, cont'd  D,** Same radiograph as **A.**

 1. First incisor tooth (*dentes incisivi*)
 2. Second incisor tooth (*dentes incisivi*)
 3. Third incisor tooth (*dentes incisivi*)
 4. Alveolar margin, interdental (*margo interalveolaris*)
 5. Alveolar margin, labial (*margo alveolaris*)
 6. Alveolar margin, palatal (*margo alveolaris*)
 7. Cervical burn-out
 8. Coronal enamel (accentuated due to tangential effect)
 9. Crown margin—palatal
10. Dentin (*dentinum*)
11. Incisive bone, nasal process (*os incisivum, processus nasalis*)
12. Incisive canal (*canalis incisivus*)
13. Incisivomaxillary suture (*sutura incisivomaxillaris*)
14. Interdental alveolar septum (*septa interalveolaria*)
15. Interincisive suture (*sutura interincisiva*)
16. Maxilla
17. Nasal bone (*os nasale*)
18. Nasal ridge of incisive bone
19. Palatine fissure (*fissura palatina*)
20. Periodontal ligament space (*periodontium, articulatio dentoalveolaris*)
21. Pulp chamber (*cavum coronale dentis, pulpa coronalis*)
22. Root canal (*canalis radicis dentis, pulpa radicularis*)
23. Vomer

## MAXILLARY INCISOR TEETH

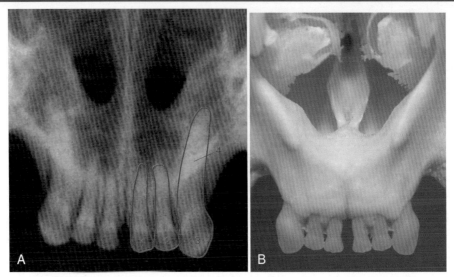

**FIGURE 3-2 Normal incisor teeth in adult cat.** Superimposition of the nasal ridge of the incisive bone over the incisor roots has been shifted apically (compared to Figure 3.3.1) by angulation of the x-ray beam (ventral tube shift) to elongate the incisor roots. **A,** Radiograph of incisors in adult cat skull. **B,** Dorsal view of prepared skull
1. First incisor tooth (*dentes incisivi*)
2. Second incisor tooth (*dentes incisivi*)
3. Third incisor tooth (*dentes incisivi*)
4. Nasal ridge of incisive bone

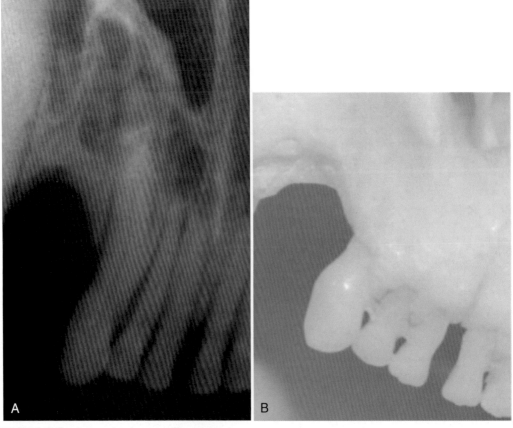

**FIGURE 3-3** For legend see opposite page.

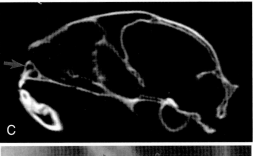

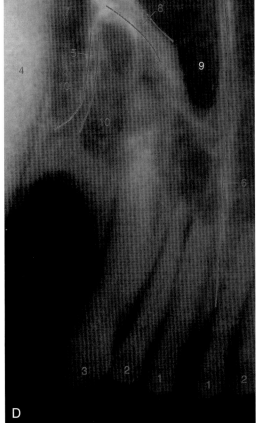

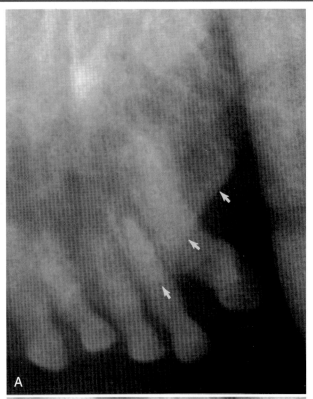

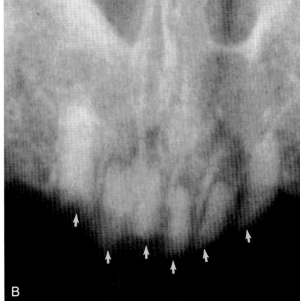

**FIGURE 3-3** The maxillary third incisor tooth and interalveolar bone (between third incisor and canine) can be better imaged using a more lateral projection angle. **A,** (facing page) Radiograph of adult cat skull. **B,** (facing page) Labial view of prepared cat skull. **C,** Saggital plane from CT image of cat skull at level of maxillary third incisor. Area of hypoattenuation in the periapical area (*arrow*) corresponds to area of decreased bone density around the root tip of the maxillary third incisor. **D,** Same radiograph as in **A.**

1. First incisor tooth (*dentes incisivi*)
2. Second incisor tooth (*dentes incisivi*)
3. Third incisor tooth (*dentes incisivi*)
4. Canine tooth (*dentes canini*)
5. Incisivomaxillary suture (*sutura incisivomaxillaris*)
6. Interincisive suture (*sutura interincisiva*)
7. Maxilla
8. Nasal ridge of incisive bone (*os incisivum*)
9. Palatine fissure
10. Trabecular bone

**FIGURE 3-4** Radiographs demonstrating dental problems. **A,** Periodontal disease (periodontitis) with associated alveolar bone loss (*arrows*). **B,** Radiograph of rostral maxilla revealing six retained roots (*arrows*) from a cat "missing" all the incisors.

## MAXILLARY CANINE TEETH

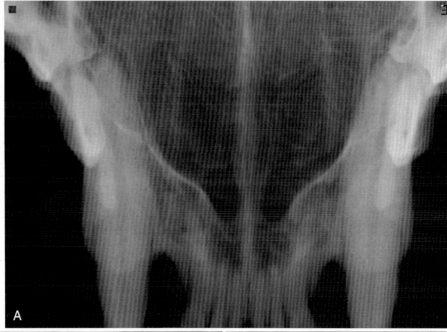

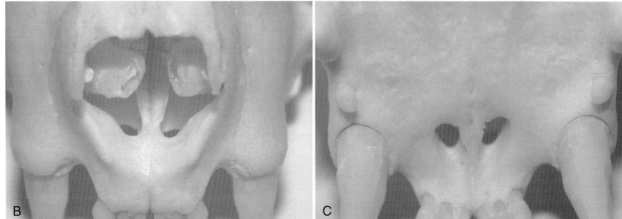

FIGURE 3-5 **Normal adult cat canine teeth. A,** Radiograph of the skull of an adult cat showing the canine teeth and surrounding structures. **B,** Dorsal view of prepared skull. **C,** Ventral (mirror) view of skull.

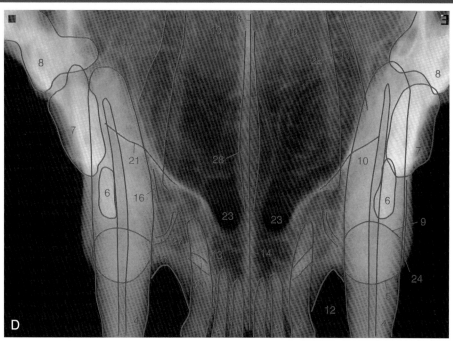

FIGURE 3-5, cont'd **D**, Same radiograph as **A.**

1. First incisor tooth (*dentes incisivi*)
2. Second incisor tooth (*dentes incisivi*)
3. Third incisor tooth (*dentes incisivi*)
4. Canine tooth (*dentes canini*)
5. Alveolar margin, buccal (*margo alveolaris*)
6. Second premolar tooth (*dentes premolares*)
7. Third premolar tooth (*dentes premolares*)
8. Fourth premolar tooth (*dentes premolares*)
9. Alveolar margin, palatal (*margo alveolaris*)
10. Dentin (*dentinum*)
11. Incisive bone, nasal process (*os incisivum, processus nasalis*)
12. Interalveolar margin (*margo interalveolaris*)
13. Interalveolar septum (*septa interalveolaria*)
14. Interincisive suture (*sutura interincisiva*)
15. Incisivomaxillary suture (*sutura incisivomaxillaris*)
16. Lamina dura
17. Maxilla
18. Median palatal suture (*sutura palatina mediana*)
19. Nasal bone (*os nasale*)
20. Nasal ridge of incisive bone (*os incisivum*)
21. Nasal surface of alveolar process of maxilla (*facies nasalis, processus alveolaris*)
22. Nasoincisive suture (*sutura nasoincisiva*)
23. Palatine fissure (*fissura palatina*)
24. Periodontal ligament space (*periodontium, articulatio dentoalveolaris*)
25. Pulp chamber (*cavum coronale dentis, pulpa coronalis*)
26. Root canal (*canalis radicis dentis, pulpa radicularis*)
27. Trabecular bone (*substantia spongiosa ossium*)
28. Vomer

## MAXILLARY CANINE TEETH

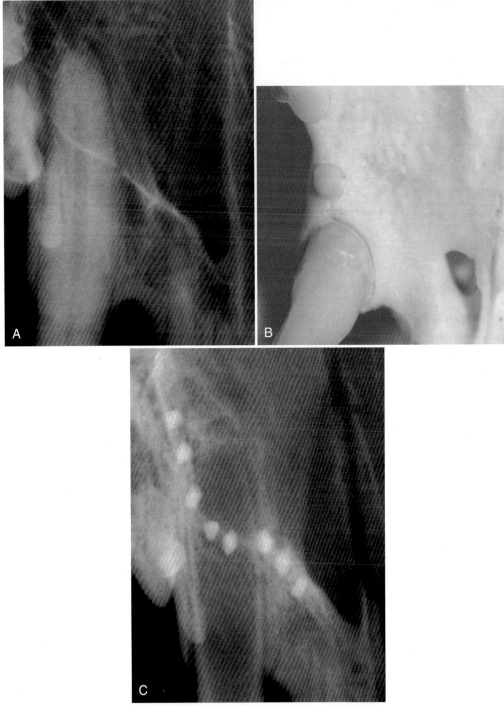

**FIGURE 3-6 Normal adult cat canine tooth. A,** Radiograph of the maxillary right canine tooth. **B,** Palatal view of prepared skull specimen. **C,** Radiograph illustrating the nasal surface of the alveolar process of the maxilla. Holes were drilled into the nasal surface of the maxilla bone where the nasal and palatal portions meet and these were filled with gutta percha.

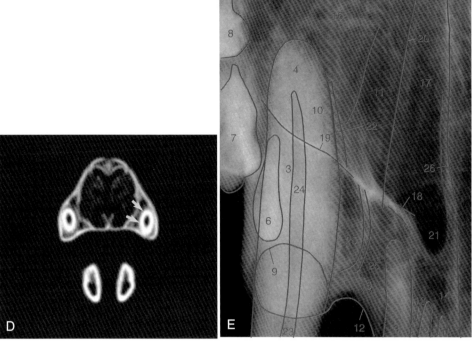

**FIGURE 3-6, cont'd   D,** CT scan, transverse plane at mid-root of canine teeth (arrows). **E,** Same radiograph as in **A.**

1. First incisor tooth (*dentes incisivi*)
2. Second incisor tooth (*dentes incisivi*)
3. Third incisor tooth (*dentes incisivi*)
4. Canine tooth (*dentes canini*)
5. Alveolar margin, labial (*margo alveolaris*)
6. Second premolar tooth (*dentes premolares*)
7. Third premolar tooth (*dentes premolares*)
8. Fourth premolar tooth (*dentes premolares*)
9. Alveolar margin, palatal (*margo alveolaris*)
10. Dentin (*dentinum*)
11. Incisive bone, nasal process (*os incisivum, processus nasalis*)
12. Interalveolar margin (*margo interalveolaris*)
13. Interalveolar septum (*septa interalveolaria*)
14. Interincisive suture (*sutura interincisiva*)
15. Incisivomaxillary suture (*sutura incisivomaxillaris*)
16. Maxilla
17. Nasal bone (*os nasale*)
18. Nasal ridge of incisive bone (*os incisivum*)
19. Nasal surface of alveolar process of maxilla (*facies nasalis, processus alveolaris*)
20. Nasoincisive suture (*sutura nasoincisiva*)
21. Palatine fissure (*fissura palatina*)
22. Periodontal ligament space (*periodontium, articulatio dentoalveolaris*)
23. Pulp chamber (*cavum coronale dentis, pulpa coronalis*)
24. Root canal (*canalis radicis dentis, pulpa radicularis*)
25. Trabecular bone (*substantia spongiosa ossium*)
26. Vomer

## MAXILLARY CANINE TEETH

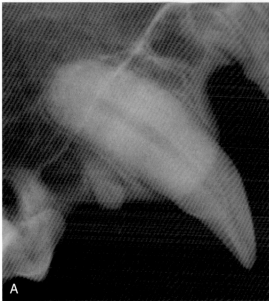

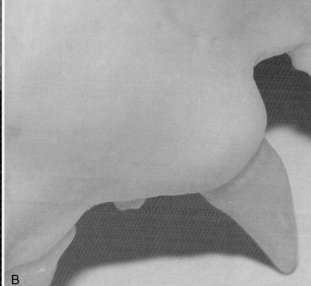

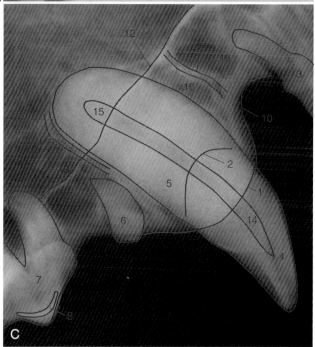

FIGURE 3-7 **A,** Radiograph of the right canine tooth and surrounding structures in an adult cat. **B,** Labial view of prepared specimen. **C,** Same radiograph as in **A.**

1. Alveolar margin, labial (*margo alveolaris*)
2. Alveolar margin, palatal (*margo alveolaris*)
3. Third incisor tooth (*dentes incisivi*)
4. Canine tooth (*dentes canini*)
5. Dentin (*dentinum*)
6. Second premolar tooth (*dentes premolares*)
7. Third premolar tooth (*dentes premolares*)
8. Enamel (*enamelum*)
9. Incisivomaxillary suture (*sutura incisivomaxillaris*)
10. Interalveolar margin (*margo interalveolaris*)
11. Lamina dura (*alveoli dentales*)
12. Nasal surface of alveolar process of maxilla (*facies nasalis, processus alveolaris*)
13. Periodontal ligament space (*periodontium, articulatio dentoalveolaris*)
14. Pulp chamber (*cavum coronale dentis, pulpa coronalis*)
15. Root canal (*canalis radicis dentis, pulpa radicularis*)
16. Trabecular bone (*substantia spongiosa ossium*)

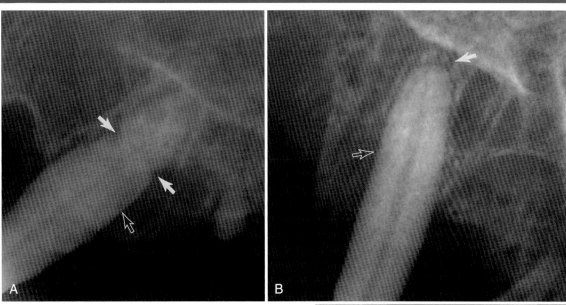

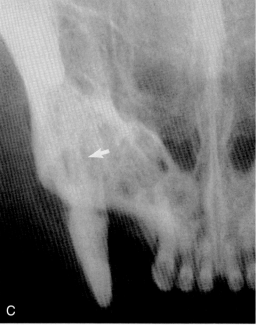

**FIGURE 3-8** Radiographs of feline canine teeth demonstrating commonly found abnormalities. **A,** Radiograph of the left maxillary canine tooth in an adult cat demonstrating severe alveolar (attachment) bone loss (*open arrow*) and external root resorption (*arrow*) associated with severe periodontitis. **B,** Radiograph of right maxillary canine revealing loss of apical lamina dura (*arrow*) (endodontic disease, see Chapter 6) and alveolar bone loss (*open arrow*) (periodontitis, see Chapter 5). **C,** Radiograph of maxillary right canine revealing severe root resorption (*arrow*) typically seen with tooth resorption in feline canine teeth (see Chapter 7).

## MAXILLARY PREMOLAR AND MOLAR TEETH

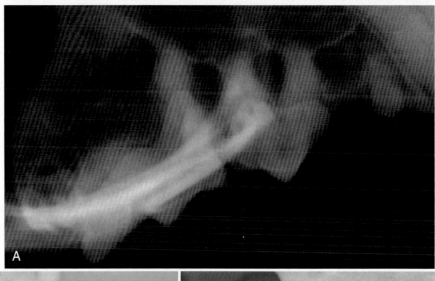

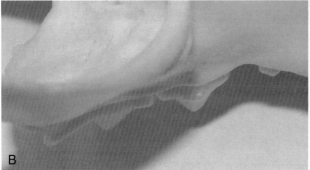

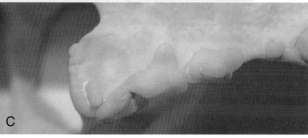

**FIGURE 3-9 Normal maxillary premolar and molar teeth in the adult cat.** The premolar and molar teeth are all within the alveolar process of the maxilla. Radiographs of the maxillary premolar and molar teeth in cats often projects through the zygomatic bone. **A,** Radiograph of the right maxillary premolar and molar region of an adult cat skull. **B,** Buccal (vestibular) view of prepared adult cat skull. **C,** Palatal view of maxillary premolars and molar in a prepared skull.

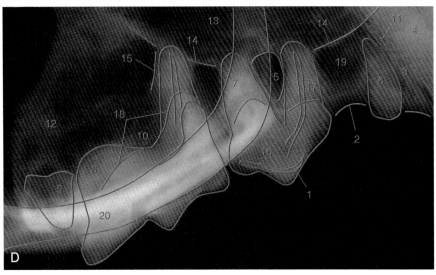

FIGURE 3-9, cont'd  **D,** Same radiograph as **A.**

1. Coronal enamel (*enamelum*)
2. Interalveolar margin (*margo interalveolaris*)
3. Interdental alveolar septum (*septa interradicularia*)
4. Canine tooth (*dentes canini*)
5. Infraorbital canal (*canalis infraorbitalis*)
6. Second premolar tooth (*dentes premolares*)
7. Third premolar tooth (*dentes premolares*)
8. Fourth premolar tooth (*dentes premolares*)
9. First molar tooth (*dentes molars*)
10. Interradicular bone (*septa interradicularia*)
11. Lamina dura—compact bone of alveolar wall (*alveoli dentales*)
12. Maxillary tuberosity (*tuber maxillae*)
13. Nasal cavity (*cavum nasi*)
14. Nasal surface of alveolar process of maxilla (*facies nasalis, processus alveolaris*)
15. Periodontal ligament space (*periodontium, articulatio dentoalveolaris*)
16. Pulp chamber (*cavum coronale dentis, pulpa coronalis*)
17. Root canal (*canalis radicis dentis, pulpa radicularis*)
18. Tooth crowns—premolars
19. Trabecular bone (*substantia spongiosa ossium*)
20. Zygomatic bone (*os zygomaticum*)

## MAXILLARY PREMOLAR AND MOLAR TEETH

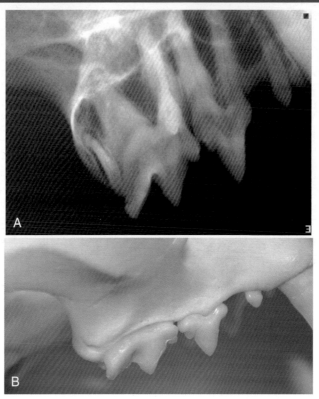

**FIGURE 3-10** Shifting the direction of the x-ray beam to a more horizontal projection moves the zygomatic bone apically. This projection may be used to evaluate the crowns, furcation area, and coronal portions of the roots. **A,** Radiograph of maxillary premolars and molar. **B,** Buccal view of the maxillary premolars and molar in a prepared skull.

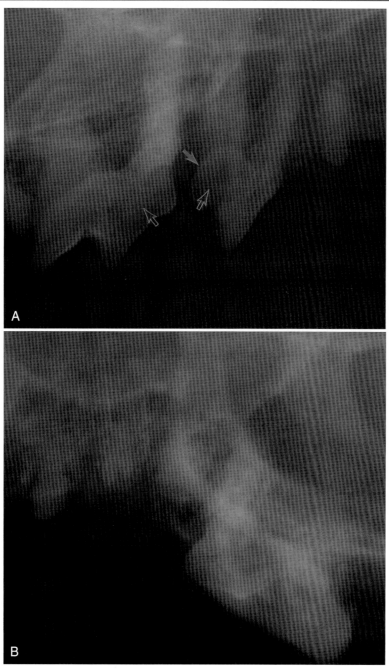

**FIGURE 3-11  Common pathology. A,** Bone loss (*arrow*) from periodontal disease (see Chapter 5) and tooth resorption (see Chapter 7) affecting the third and fourth premolars (*open arrows*). **B,** Persistent roots of the third premolar (*arrows*).

## MANDIBULAR INCISOR TEETH

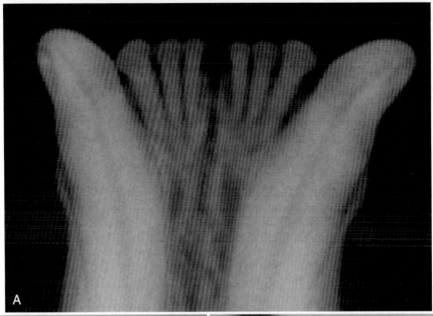

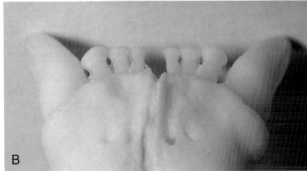

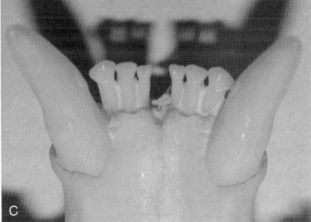

FIGURE 3-12 Mandibular incisor teeth. **A,** Radiograph of the incisor teeth and rostral mandibular region of a mature cat. **B,** Ventral view of rostral mandibles from a prepared skull. **C,** Dorsal (mirror image) view of the rostral mandibles.

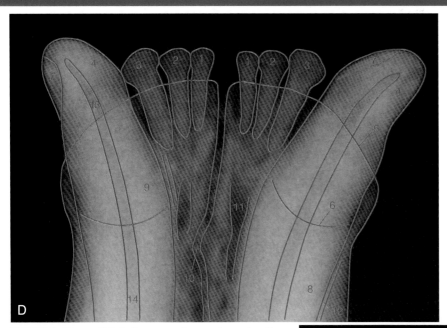

**FIGURE 3-12, cont'd  D,** Same radiograph as **A** with structures labeled. **E,** Transverse plane image of CT scan at level of mandibular incisors.

1. First incisor tooth (*dentes incisivi*)
2. Second incisor tooth (*dentes incisivi*)
3. Third incisor tooth (*dentes incisivi*)
4. Canine tooth (*dentes canini*)
5. Alveolar bone margin—labial (*margo alveolaris*)
6. Alveolar bone margin—lingual (*margo alveolaris*)
7. Coronal enamel (accentuated due to tangential effect) (*enamelum*)
8. Dentin (*dentinum*)
9. Lamina dura (*alveoli dentales*)
10. Mandibular symphysis (*synchondrosis intermandibularis*)
11. Nutrient canal
12. Periodontal ligament space (*periodontium, articulatio dentoalveolaris*)
13. Pulp chamber (*cavum coronale dentis, pulpa coronalis*)
14. Root canal (*canalis radicis dentis, pulpa radicularis*)

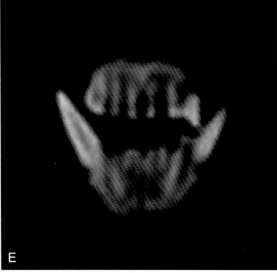

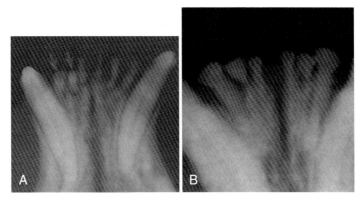

**FIGURE 3-13  Adult cat with severe periodontitis and bone loss.  A,** The mandibular right second and third incisors were very mobile and not in the normal position (*arrow*). **B,** Adult cat with tooth resorption (Type 1) of the mandibular second incisors.

## MANDIBULAR CANINE TEETH

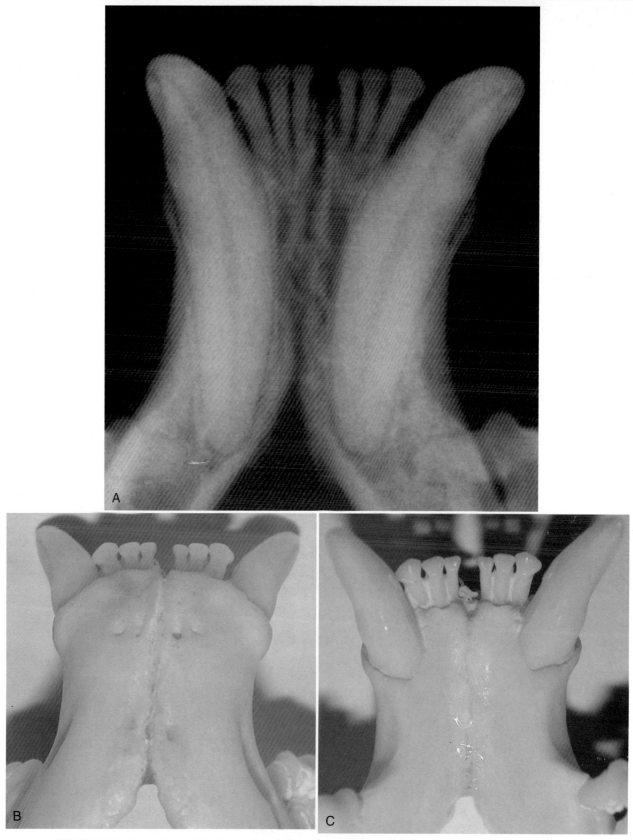

FIGURE 3-14 Normal mandibular canine teeth in adult cat. **A,** Radiograph of the rostral mandibles from an adult cat showing the canine teeth and surrounding structures. **B,** Labial view of prepared mandibles. **C,** Lingual (mirror image view) of the mandibles.

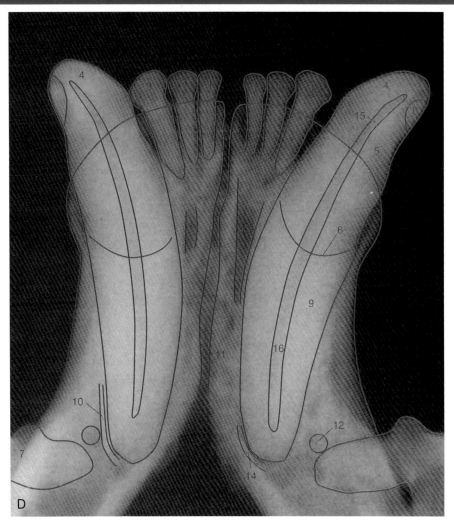

**FIGURE 3-14, cont'd  D,** Same radiograph as **A.**

1. First incisor tooth (*dentes incisivi*)
2. Second incisor tooth (*dentes incisivi*)
3. Third incisor tooth (*dentes incisivi*)
4. Canine tooth (*dentes canini*)
5. Alveolar margin—labial (*margo alveolaris*)
6. Alveolar margin—lingual (*margo alveolaris*)
7. Third premolar tooth (*dentes premolares*)
8. Coronal enamel (*enamelum*)
9. Dentin (*dentinum*)
10. Lamina dura (*alveoli dentales*)
11. Mandibular symphysis (*synchondrosis intermandibularis*)
12. Mental foramen, middle (*foramen mentale*)
13. Nutrient canal
14. Periodontal ligament space (*periodontium, articulatio dentoalveolaris*)
15. Pulp chamber (*cavum coronale dentis, pulpa coronalis*)
16. Root canal (*canalis radicis dentis, pulpa radicularis*)

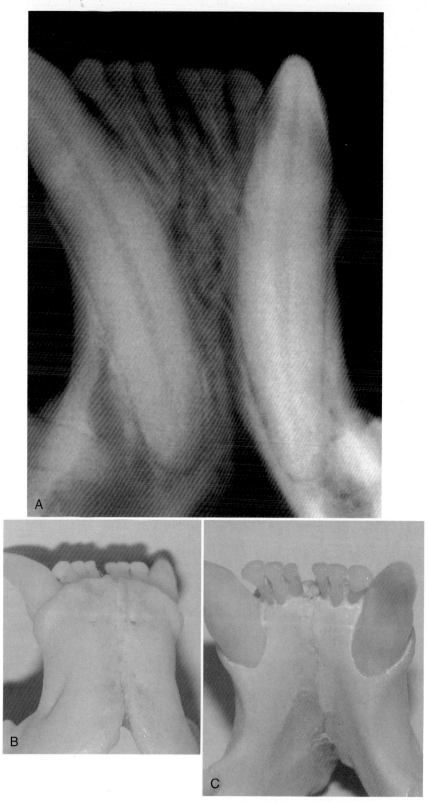

FIGURE 3-15 An oblique radiographic view of the right mandibular canine tooth in an adult cat skull. **A,** Right canine tooth and surrounding structures. **B,** Labial view of prepared mandibles. **C,** Lingual (mirror image) view of mandibles.

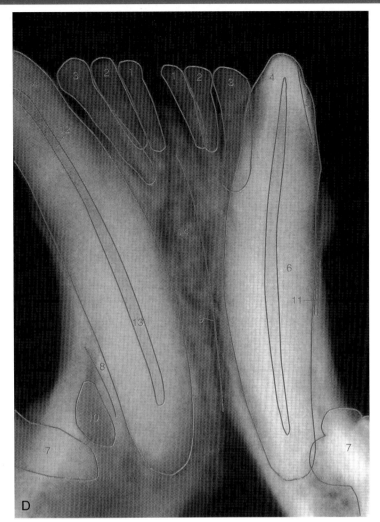

**FIGURE 3-15, cont'd  D,** Same radiograph as **A.**

1. First incisor tooth (*dentes incisivi*)
2. Second incisor tooth (*dentes incisivi*)
3. Third incisor tooth (*dentes incisivi*)
4. Canine tooth (*dentes canini*)
5. Coronal enamel (visible due to tangential effect)
6. Dentin (*dentinum*)
7. Third premolar tooth (*dentes premolares*)
8. Lamina dura (*alveoli dentales*)
9. Mandibular symphysis (*synchondrosis intermandibularis*)
10. Mental foramen—middle (*foramen mentale*)
11. Periodontal ligament space (*periodontium, articulatio dentoalveolaris*)
12. Pulp chamber (*cavum coronale dentis, pulpa coronalis*)
13. Root canal (*canalis radicis dentis, pulpa radicularis*)
14. Trabecular bone (*substantia spongiosa ossium*)

## MANDIBULAR CANINE TEETH

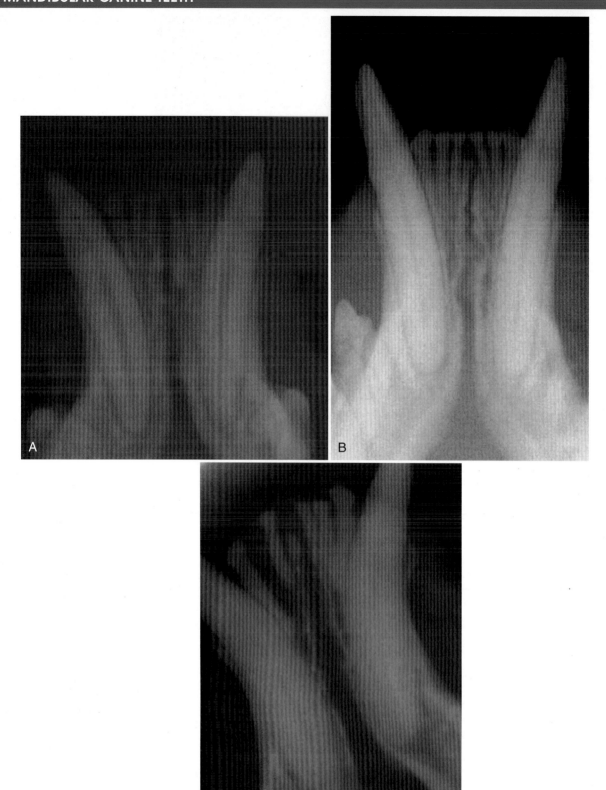

FIGURE 3-16 **Mandibular symphysis in cats. A,** Mandibular symphysis in a young adult cat. **B,** Mandibular symphysis in an older adult cat, **C,** Separation of the mandibular symphysis in an adult cat secondary to trauma.

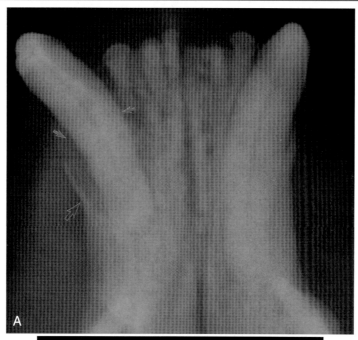

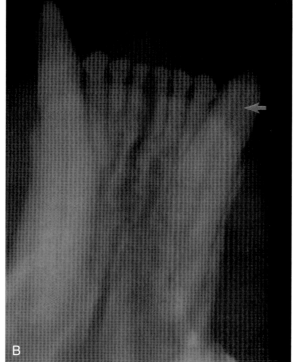

**FIGURE 3-17 Commonly found pathology. A,** Periodontitis. Horizontal and vertical alveolar bone loss (*arrow*) with alveolar bony expansion of the right canine tooth (*open arrow*) (see Chapter 5). **B,** Endodontic disease of left canine tooth (*arrow*) secondary to an open fracture. Wider root canal of left canine compared to the right canine. Apical root resorption may occur as a result of chronic endodontic disease (see Chapter 6).

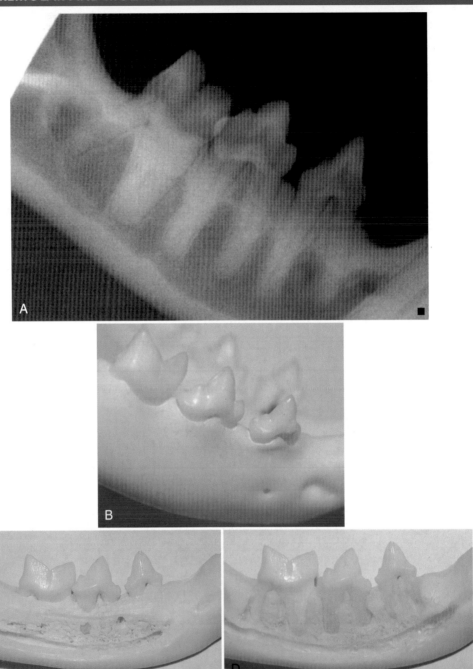

**FIGURE 3-18** Normal mandibular premolar and molar teeth in adult cat. **A,** Radiograph of the right mandibular premolar and molar teeth of an adult feline skull. **B,** Buccal view of a prepared mandible. **C,** Prepared specimen with partial removal of mandibular buccal compact and trabecular bone illustrating the ventrolateral location of the mandibular canal. **D,** Prepared specimen with complete removal of mandibular buccal bone exposing the mandibular tooth roots and canal.

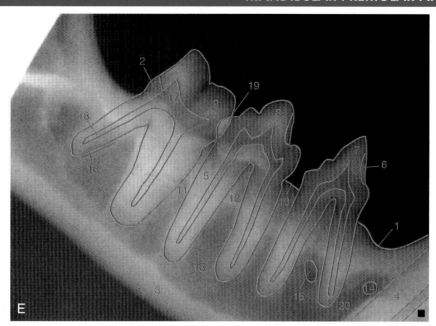

**FIGURE 3-18, cont'd E,** Same radiograph as **A.**

1. Alveolar margin interdental (*margo interalveolaris*)
2. Cervical burn-out caused by a relative lack of superimposed structures
3. Compact bone of ventral mandible (*margo ventralis*)
4. Canine tooth (*dentes canini*)
5. Dentin (*dentinum*)
6. Enamel (*enamelum*)
7. Third premolar tooth (*dentes premolares*)
8. Fourth premolar tooth (*dentes premolares*)
9. First molar tooth (*dentes molares*)
10. Interalveolar margin (*margo interalveolaris*)
11. Interdental alveolar septum (*septa interalveolaria*)
12. Interradicular bone (*septa interradicularia*)
13. Mandibular canal (*canalis mandibulae*)
14. Mental foramen, middle (*foramina mentalia*)
15. Mental foramen, caudal (*foramina mentalia*)
16. Periodontal ligament space (*periodontium, articulatio dentoalveolari*)
17. Pulp chamber (*cavum coronale dentis, pulpa coronalis*)
18. Root canal (*canalis radicis dentis, pulpa radicularis*)
19. Superimposition of proximal contacts
20. Trabecular bone (*substantia spongiosa ossium*)

## MANDIBULAR PREMOLAR AND MOLAR TEETH

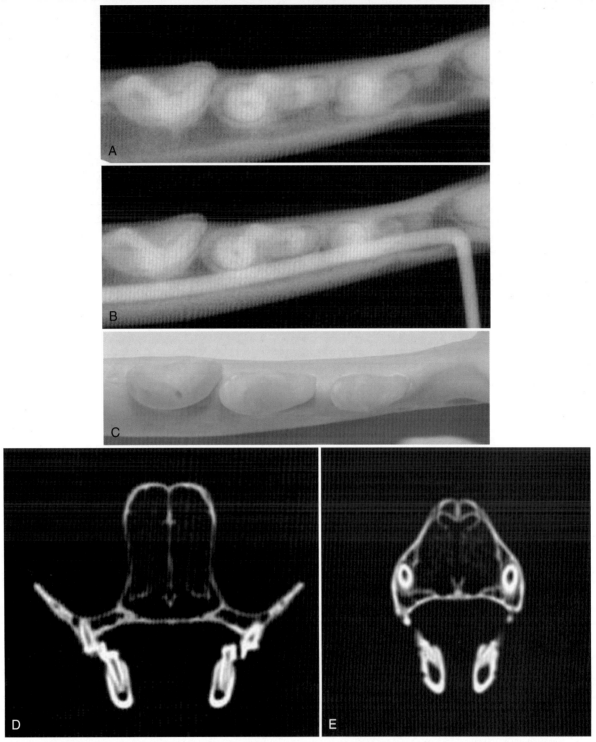

**FIGURE 3-19  Right mandible in an adult cat. A,** The buccal–lingual orientation of the premolars and molar in the mandible is shown. **B,** Gutta percha point entering into the mandibular canal through the middle mental foramen illustrating the lateral position of the mandibular canal. **C,** Occlusal view of right mandible from prepared skull. **D,** Transverse plane image of CT scan at the level of the mesial root of the mandibular molar demonstrating the ventral position of the mandibular canal. **E,** Transverse plane image of CT scan at the level of the mesial root of the mandibular third premolar demonstrating the ventrolateral position of the mandibular canal.

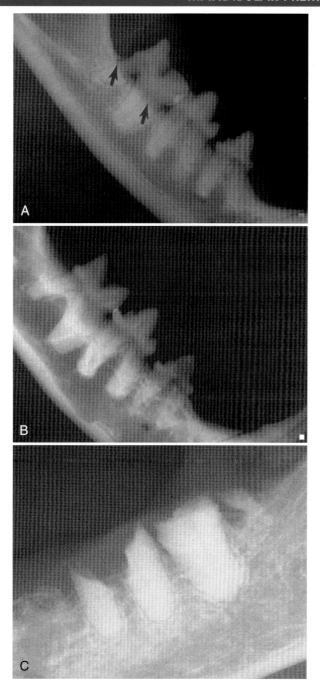

**FIGURE 3-20 Common dental problems. A,** Horizontal bone loss (*arrow*) from periodontitis (see Chapter 5). **B,** Type 2 tooth resorption of right third premolar (see Chapter 7). **C,** Retained roots associated with soft tissue inflammation.

## NORMAL TEETH IN THE KITTEN

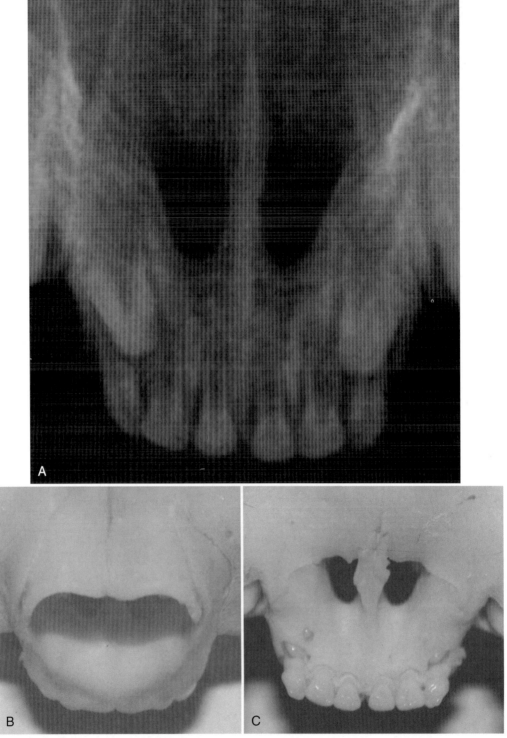

**FIGURE 3-21** Normal deciduous and permanent maxillary incisor teeth in a kitten in the mixed dentition stage. **A,** Radiograph of the incisor teeth and rostral maxillary region of a kitten with a mixed dentition. **B,** Dorsal view of prepared skull. **C,** Ventral (mirror image) view of skull.

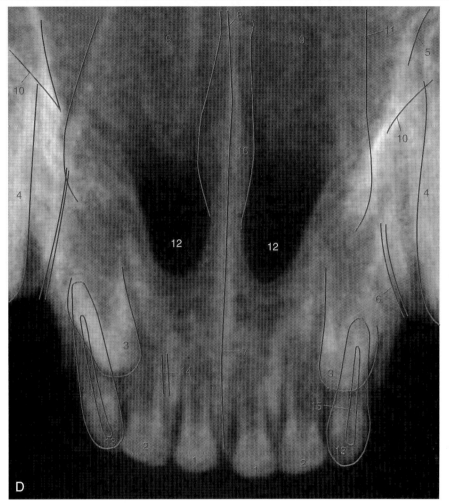

**FIGURE 3-21, cont'd  D,** Same radiograph as **A.** The roots of the deciduous third incisors are positioned labial to the developing permanent teeth.

1. Permanent first incisor tooth (*dentes permanentes, dentes incisivi*)
2. Permanent second incisor tooth (*dentes permanentes, dentes incisivi*)
3. Permanent third incisor tooth (*dentes permanentes, dentes incisivi*)
4. Canine tooth (*dentes canini*)
5. Bony crypt of permanent tooth follicle
6. Incisivomaxillary suture (*sutura incisivomaxillaris*)
7. Interincisive suture (*sutura interincisiva*)
8. Median palatal suture (*sutura palatine mediana*)
9. Nasal bone (*os nasale*)
10. Nasal surface of alveolar process of maxilla (*facies nasalis, processus alveolaris*)
11. Nasoincisive suture (*sutura nasoincisiva*)
12. Palatine fissure (*fissura palatina*)
13. Deciduous third incisor tooth (*dentes decidui, dentes incisivi*)
14. Periodontal ligament space (*periodontium, articulatio dentoalveolari*)
15. Root canal (*canalis radicis dentis, pulpa radicularis*)
16. Vomer

## NORMAL TEETH IN THE KITTEN

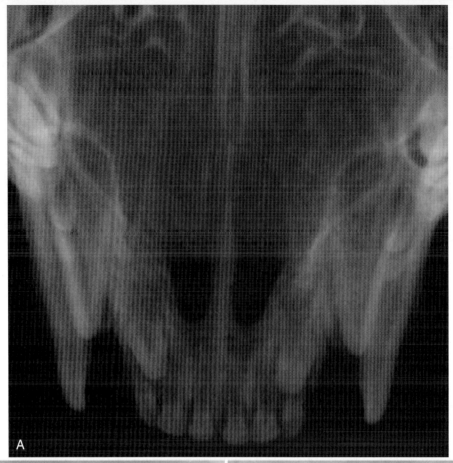

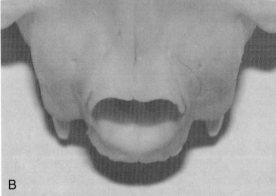

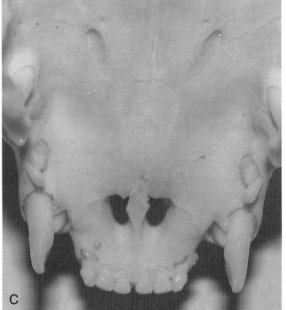

**FIGURE 3-22** **Normal deciduous maxillary canine teeth.** **A,** Radiograph of the maxillary canine teeth of a kitten in the mixed dentition stage. **B,** Dorsal view of prepared skull. **C,** Ventral (mirror image) view of skull.

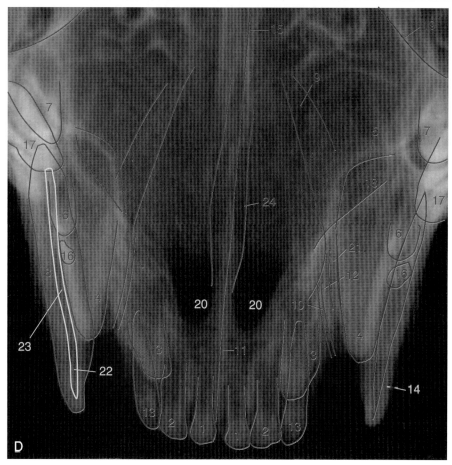

**FIGURE 3-22, cont'd  D,** Same radiograph as **A.**

1. Permanent first incisor tooth (*dentes permanentes, dentes incisivi*)
2. Permanent second incisor tooth (*dentes permanentes, dentes incisivi*)
3. Permanent third incisor tooth (*dentes permanentes, dentes incisivi*)
4. Permanent canine tooth (*dentes permanentes, dentes canini*)
5. Bony crypt of permanent tooth follicle
6. Permanent second premolar tooth (*dentes permanentes, dentes premolares*)
7. Permanent third premolar tooth (*dentes permanentes, dentes premolares*)
8. Dentin (*dentinum*)
9. Incisive bone—nasal process (*os incisivum, processus nasalis*)
10. Incisivomaxillary suture (*sutura incisivomaxillaris*)
11. Interincisive suture (*sutura interincisiva*)
12. Maxilla
13. Deciduous third incisor tooth (*dentes decidui, dentes incisivi*)
14. Deciduous canine tooth (*dentes decidui, dentes canini*)
15. Median palatal suture (*sutura palatine mediana*)
16. Deciduous second premolar tooth (*dentes decidui, dentes premolares*)
17. Deciduous third premolar tooth (*dentes decidui, dentes premolares*)
18. Nasal surface of alveolar process of maxilla (*facies nasalis, processus alveolaris*)
19. Orbital rim (*os zygomaticum, margo infraorbitalis*)
20. Palatine fissure (*fissura palatina*)
21. Periodontal ligament space (*periodontium, articulatio dentoalveolari*)
22. Pulp chamber (*cavum coronale dentis, pulpa coronalis*)
23. Root canal (*canalis radicis dentis, pulpa radicularis*)
24. Vomer

## NORMAL TEETH IN THE KITTEN

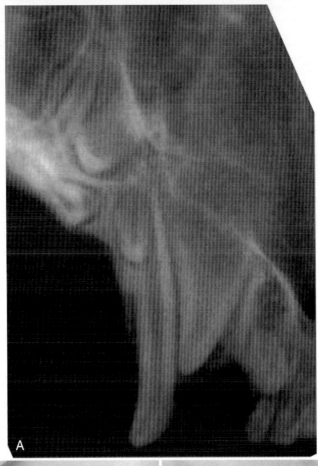

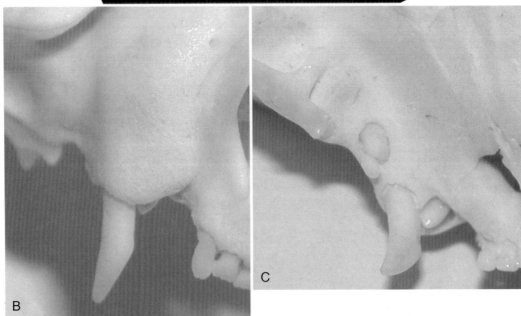

**FIGURE 3-23** **Normal deciduous canine tooth. A,** Radiograph of the canine tooth and surrounding structures of a kitten in the mixed dentition stage. **B,** Labial view of prepared skull. **C,** Palatal (mirror image) view of skull.

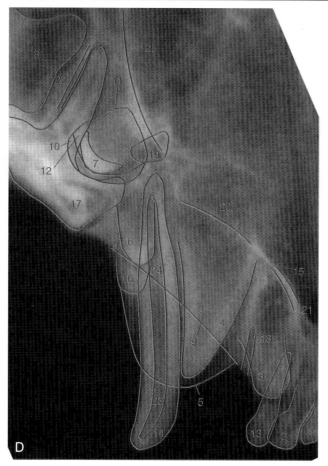

**FIGURE 3-23, cont'd  D,** Same radiograph as **A.** The underlying successor permanent second premolar tooth is superimposed over the deciduous canine tooth root. The palatal surface of the maxillary bone is operculated at future eruption sites. The majority of the radiolucency coronal to the developing crowns is a result of the eruption cyst, a normal part of the eruption process.

1. Permanent first incisor tooth (*dentes permanentes, dentes incisivi*)
2. Permanent second incisor tooth (*dentes permanentes, dentes incisivi*)
3. Permanent third incisor tooth (*dentes permanentes, dentes incisivi*)
4. Permanent canine tooth (*dentes permanentes, dentes canini*)
5. Alveolar margin—buccal (*margo alveolaris*)
6. Permanent second premolar tooth (*dentes permanentes, dentes premolares*)
7. Permanent third premolar tooth (*dentes permanentes, dentes premolares*)
8. Permanent fourth premolar tooth (*dentes permanentes, dentes premolares*)
9. Alveolar margin—palatal (*margo alveolaris*)
10. Bony crypt of permanent tooth follicle
11. Dental follicle
12. Eruption cyst
13. Deciduous third incisor tooth (*dentes decidui, dentes incisivi*)
14. Deciduous canine tooth (*dentes decidui, dentes canini*)
15. Nasal ridge—incisive bone (*os incisivum*)
16. Deciduous second premolar tooth (*dentes decidui, dentes premolares*)
17. Deciduous third premolar tooth (*dentes decidui, dentes premolares*)
18. Incisivomaxillary suture (*sutura incisivomaxillaris*)
19. Infraorbital foramen (*foramen infraorbitale*)
20. Nasal surface of alveolar process of maxilla (*facies nasalis, processus alveolaris*)
21. Palatine fissure (*fissura palatina*)
22. Periodontal ligament space (*periodontium, articulatio dentoalveolari*)
23. Pulp chamber (*cavum coronale dentis, pulpa coronalis*)
24. Root canal (*canalis radicis dentis, pulpa radicularis*)
25. Zygomatic bone (*os zygomaticum*)

## NORMAL TEETH IN THE KITTEN

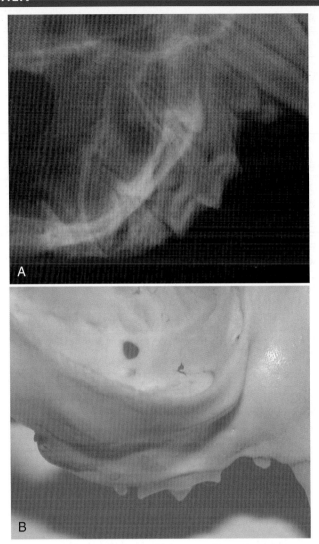

**FIGURE 3-24** Relationship of the zygomatic arch to the maxillary deciduous premolar teeth. **A** and **C,** Radiographs of the premolar teeth and surrounding structures of a kitten in the deciduous dentition stage. **B** and **D,** Buccal views of prepared skull approximating the same relationship between the premolars and zygomatic bone.

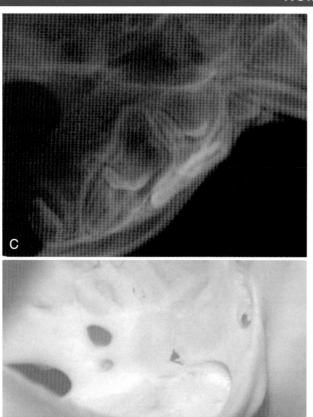

FIGURE 3-24, cont'd

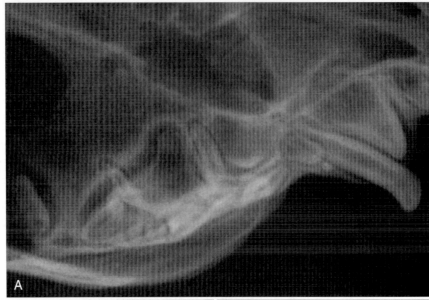

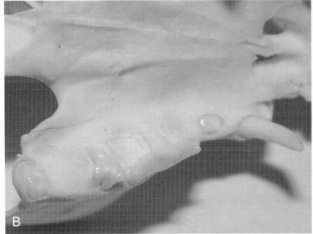

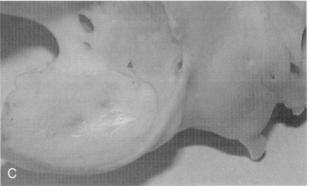

**FIGURE 3-25** Developing permanent maxillary premolar and molar teeth. **A,** Radiograph of the maxillary molar area of a kitten in the deciduous dentition stage. **B,** Palatal view of skull. **C,** Labial view of skull.

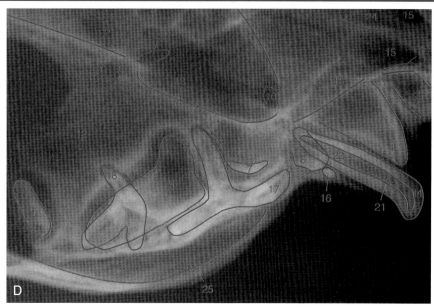

FIGURE 3-25, cont'd  **D,** Same radiograph as **A.**

1. Caudal palatine foramen (*foramen palatinum caudale*)
2. Choanae—lateral border
3. Permanent third incisor tooth (*dentes permanentes, dentes incisivi*)
4. Permanent canine tooth (*dentes permanentes, dentes canini*)
5. Nasal ridge—incisive bone (*os incisivum*)
6. Permanent second premolar tooth (*dentes permanentes, dentes premolares*)
7. Permanent third premolar tooth (*dentes permanentes, dentes premolares*)
8. Permanent fourth premolar tooth (*dentes permanentes, dentes premolares*)
9. Permanent first molar tooth (*dentes permanents, dentes molares*)
10. Lacrimal canal (*canalis lacrimalis*)
11. Maxilla—orbital surface (*facies orbitalis*)
12. Maxillary tuberosity (*tuber maxillae*)
13. Nasal surface of alveolar process of maxilla (*facies nasalis, processus alveolaris*)
14. Deciduous canine tooth (*dentes decidui, dentes canini*)
15. Palatine fissure (*fissura palatina*)
16. Deciduous second premolar tooth (*dentes decidui, dentes premolares*)
17. Deciduous third premolar tooth (*dentes decidui, dentes premolares*)
18. Deciduous fourth premolar tooth (*dentes decidui, dentes premolares*)
19. Periodontal ligament space (*periodontium, articulatio dentoalveolari*)
20. Pterygoid
21. Pulp chamber (*cavum coronale dentis, pulpa coronalis*)
22. Root canal (*canalis radicis dentis, pulpa radicularis*)
23. Sphenopalatine foramen (*foramen sphenopalatinum*)
24. Vomer
25. Zygomatic bone (*os zygomaticum*)

## NORMAL TEETH IN THE KITTEN

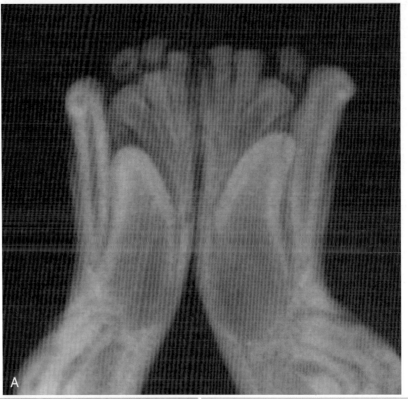

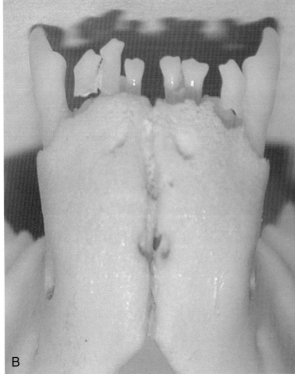

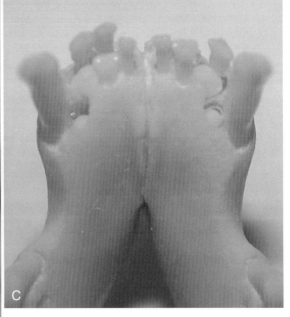

**FIGURE 3-26** Normal mandibular deciduous incisor and canine teeth. **A,** Radiograph of the incisor and canine teeth and rostral mandibles of a kitten with a mixed incisor dentition. **B,** Ventral view of prepared mandibles. **C,** Dorsal (mirror image) view of mandibles.

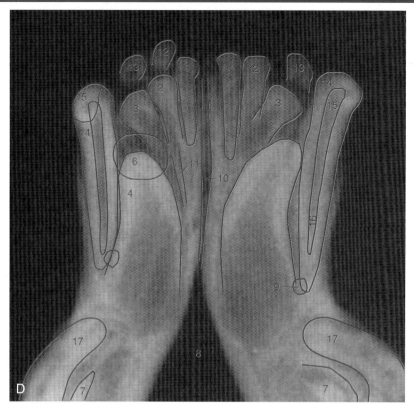

**FIGURE 3-26, cont'd D,** Same radiograph as **A.**

1. Permanent first incisor tooth (*dentes permanentes, dentes incisivi*)
2. Permanent second incisor tooth (*dentes permanentes, dentes incisivi*)
3. Permanent third incisor tooth (*dentes permanentes, dentes incisivi*)
4. Permanent canine tooth (*dentes permanentes, dentes canini*)
5. Coronal enamel (*enamelum*)
6. Gubernacular foramina
7. Permanent third premolar tooth (*dentes permanentes, dentes premolares*)
8. Intermandibular space
9. Mental foramen, middle (*foramen mentale*)
10. Mandibular symphysis (*synchondrosis intermandibularis*)
11. Nutrient canal
12. Deciduous second incisor tooth (*dentes decidui, dentes incisivi*)
13. Deciduous third incisor tooth (*dentes decidui, dentes incisivi*)
14. Deciduous canine tooth (*dentes decidui, dentes canini*)
15. Pulp chamber (*cavum coronale dentis, pulpa coronalis*)
16. Root canal (*canalis radicis dentis, pulpa radicularis*)
17. Deciduous third premolar tooth (*dentes decidui, premolares*)

## NORMAL TEETH IN THE KITTEN

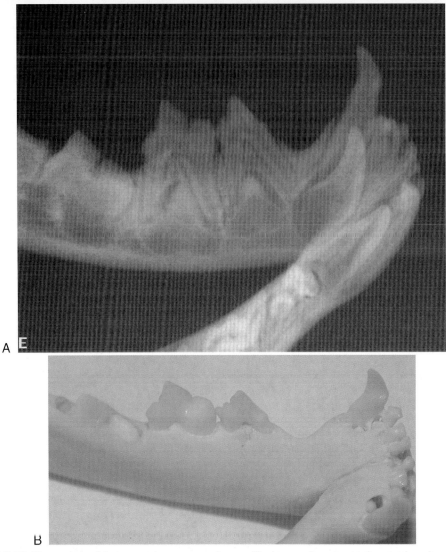

A

B

FIGURE 3-27 Normal deciduous and permanent mandibular canine, premolar, and molar teeth in a kitten in the mixed dentition stage. **A,** Radiograph of the mandibular canine, premolar, and molar teeth in a kitten in the mixed dentition stage. **B,** Lingual view of prepared skull.

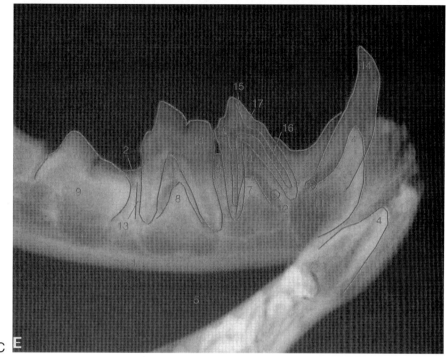

**FIGURE 3-27, cont'd C,** Same radiograph as **A.**

1. Compact bone of ventral mandible (*margo ventralis*)
2. Alveolar margin, interdental (*margo interalveolaris*)
3. Interdental alveolar septum (*septa interalveolaria*)
4. Permanent canine tooth (*dentes permanentes, dentes canini*)
5. Intermandibular space
6. Interradicular bone (*septa interradicularia*)
7. Permanent third premolar tooth (*dentes permanentes, dentes premolares*)
8. Permanent fourth premolar tooth (*dentes permanentes, dentes premolares*)
9. Permanent first molar tooth (*dentes permanentes, dentes molares*)
10. Mandibular canal (*canalis mandibulae*)
11. Mental foramen, middle (*foramen mentale*)
12. Mental foramen, caudal (*foramen mentale*)
13. Periodontal ligament space (*periodontium, articulatio dentoalveolari*)
14. Deciduous canine tooth (*dentes decidui, dentes canini*)
15. Pulp chamber (*cavum coronale dentis, pulpa coronalis*)
16. Root canal (*canalis radicis dentis, pulpa radicularis*)
17. Deciduous third premolar tooth (*dentes decidui, premolares*)
18. Deciduous fourth premolar tooth (*dentes decidui, premolares*)

# CHAPTER 4

# Temporomandibular Joint

imited imaging of the temporomandibular joint (TMJ) may be done using a dental radiograph machine and dental film or digital sensor. Skull radiographs and computed tomography images provide more information and may be necessary in many patients to adequately evaluate the TMJs. The radiographs in this section were all done using an extraoral technique with a digital sensor and dental radiograph machine.

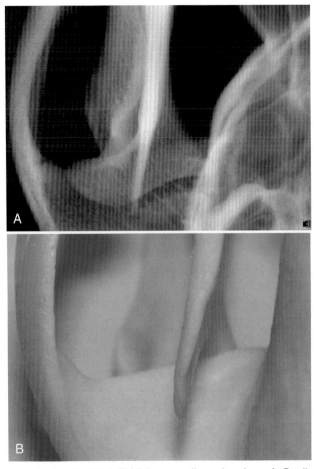

**FIGURE 4.1** Left temporomandibular joint (TMJ) in a medium-size dog. **A,** Radiograph of the left TMJ from a dog skull, dorsoventral view. **B,** Dorsal view of left TMJ from a prepared dog skull.

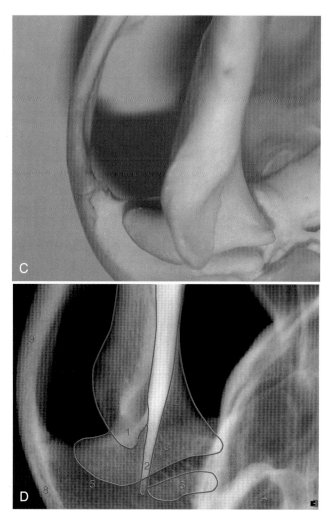

**FIGURE 4.1, cont'd C,** Ventral view (mirror) of the TMJ from a prepared dog skull. **D,** Same radiograph as **A**.

1. Angular process of mandible (*os mandibulae, processus angularis*)
2. Coronoid process of the mandible (*os mandibulae, processus coronoideus*)
3. Head of the condylar process of the mandible (*os mandibulae, processus condylaris, caput mandibulae*)
4. Neck of the condylar process of the mandible (*os mandibulae, processus condylaris, collum mandibulae*)
5. Mandibular fossa of temporal bone (*os temporal, fossa mandibularis*)
6. Retroarticular process of temporal bone (*os temporal, processus retroarticulatis*)
7. Tympanic bulla (*bulla tympanica*)
8. Zygomatic process of temporal bone (*os temporal, processus zygomaticus*)
9. Zygomatic bone (*os zygomaticum*)

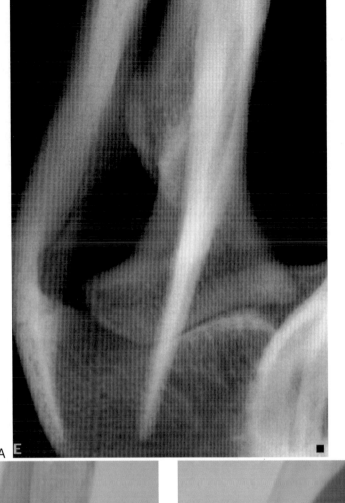

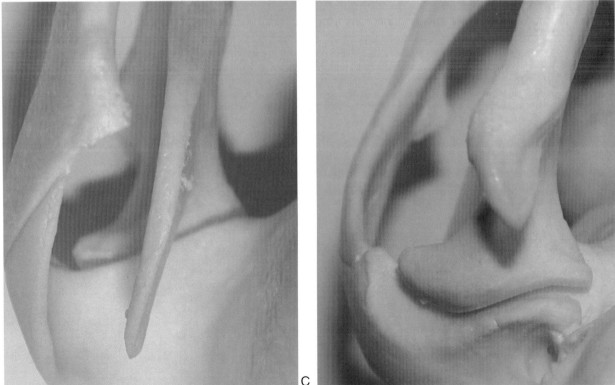

**FIGURE 4.2  Left temporomandibular joint (TMJ) in a medium-size dog.  A,** Radiograph of the left TMJ from a dog skull, intraorbital view. **B,** Dorsal view of left TMJ from a prepared dog skull. **C,** Ventral view (mirror) of the TMJ from a dog skull.

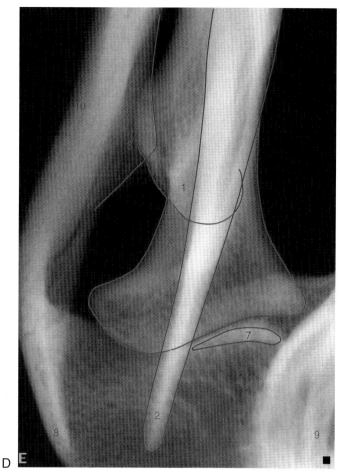

**FIGURE 4.2, cont'd  D,** Same radiograph as **A.**

1. Angular process of mandible (*os mandibulae, processus angularis*)
2. Coronoid process of the mandible (*os mandibulae, processus coronoideus*)
3. Frontal process of zygomatic bone (*os zygomaticum. processus frontalis*)
4. Head of the condylar process of the mandible (*os mandibulae, processus condylaris, caput mandibulae*)
5. Mandibular fossa of temporal bone (*os temporal, fossa mandibularis*)
6. Neck of the condylar process of the mandible (*os mandibulae, processus condylaris, collum mandibulae*)
7. Retroarticular process of temporal bone (*os temporal, processus retroarticulatis*)
8. Zygomatic process of temporal bone (*os temporal, processus zygomaticus*)
9. Tympanic bulla (*bulla tympanica*)
10. Zygomatic bone (*os zygomaticum*)

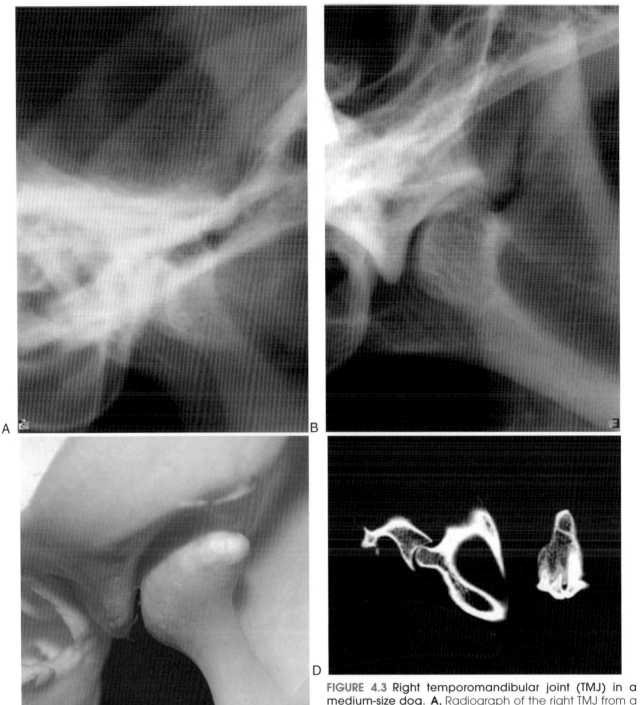

**FIGURE 4.3** Right temporomandibular joint (TMJ) in a medium-size dog. **A,** Radiograph of the right TMJ from a dog skull, laterolateral closed-mouth view. **B,** Radiograph of the right TMJ from a dog skull, lateral open-mouth view. **C,** Lateral view of right TMJ from a prepared dog skull. **D,** Transverse cut from a CT scan of a dog skull.

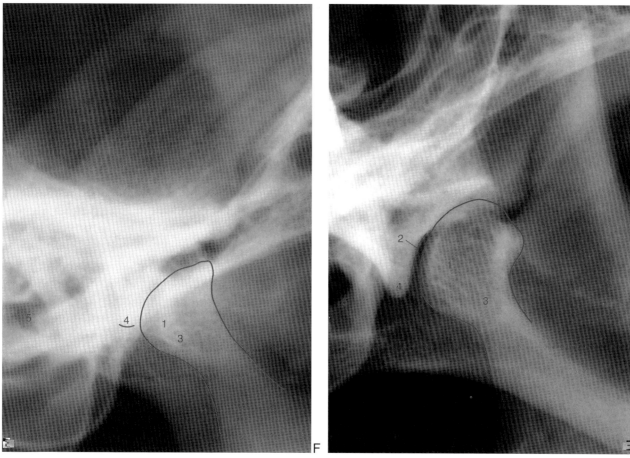

E   F

**FIGURE 4.3, cont'd  E,** Same radiograph as **A. F,** Same radiograph as **B**.

1. Head of the condylar process of the mandible (*os mandibulae, processus condylaris, caput mandibulae*)
2. Mandibular fossa of temporal bone (*os temporal, fossa mandibularis*)
3. Neck of the condylar process of the mandible (*os mandibulae, processus condylaris, collum mandibulae*)
4. Retroarticular process of temporal bone (*os temporal, processus retroarticulatis*)
5. Tympanic bulla (*bulla tympanica*)

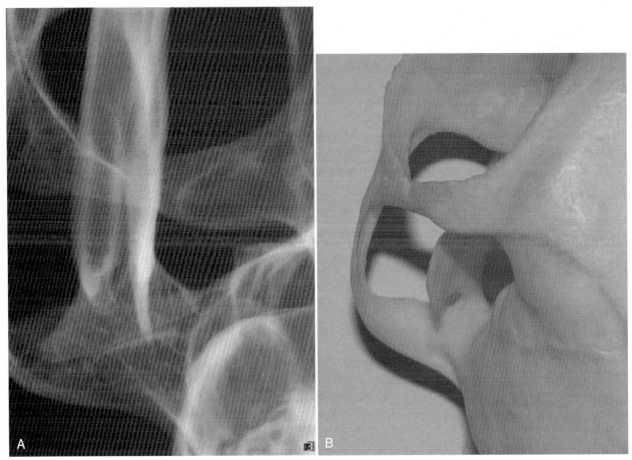

FIGURE 4.4 Left temporomandibular joint (TMJ) in a cat. **A,** Radiograph of the left TMJ from a cat skull, dorsovental view. **B,** Dorsal view of left TMJ from a prepared cat skull.

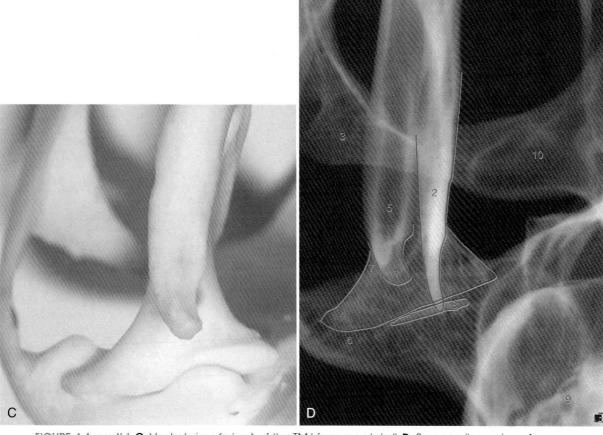

**FIGURE 4.4, cont'd C,** Ventral view (mirror) of the TMJ from a cat skull. **D,** Same radiograph as **A.**

1. Angular process of mandible (*os mandibulae, processus angularis*)
2. Coronoid process of the mandible (*os mandibulae, processus coronoideus*)
3. Frontal process of zygomatic bone (*os zygomaticum. processus frontalis*)
4. Head of the condylar process of the mandible (*os mandibulae, processus condylaris, caput mandibulae*)
5. Mandibular canal (*canalis mandibulae*)
6. Mandibular fossa of temporal bone (*os temporal, fossa mandibularis*)
7. Neck of the condylar process of the mandible (*os mandibulae, processus condylaris, collum mandibulae*)
8. Retroarticular process of temporal bone (*os temporal, processus retroarticulatis*)
9. Tympanic bulla (*bulla tympanica*)
10. Zygomatic process of frontal bone (*os frontalis, processus zygomaticus*)

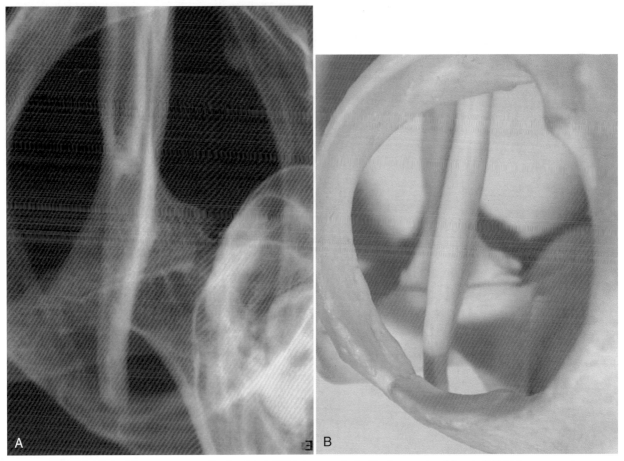

**FIGURE 4.5 Left temporomandibular joint (TMJ) in a cat. A,** Radiograph of the left TMJ from a cat skull, intraorbital view. **B,** Dorsal view of left TMJ from a prepared cat skull.

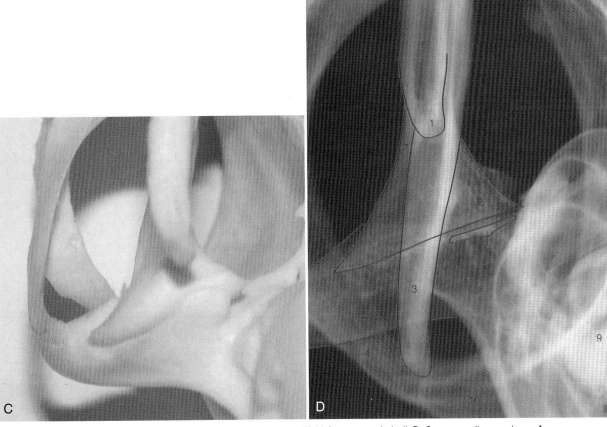

**FIGURE 4.5, cont'd  C,** Ventral view (mirror) of the TMJ from a cat skull. **D,** Same radiograph as **A.**

1. Angular process of mandible (*os mandibulae, processus angularis*)
2. Condylar process of mandible (*os mandibulae, processus condylaris, caput mandibulae*)
3. Coronoid process of mandible (*os mandibulae, processus coronoideus*)
4. Frontal process of zygomatic bone (*os zygomaticum. processus frontalis*)
5. Mandibular canal (*canalis mandibulae*)
6. Mandibular fossa of temporal bone (*os temporal, fossa mandibularis*)
7. Neck of the condylar process of the mandible (*os mandibulae, processus condylaris, collum mandibulae*)
8. Retroarticular process of temporal bone (*os temporal, processus retroarticulatis*)
9. Tympanic bulla (*bulla tympanica*)
10. Zygomatic process of frontal bone (*os frontalis, processus zygomaticus*)

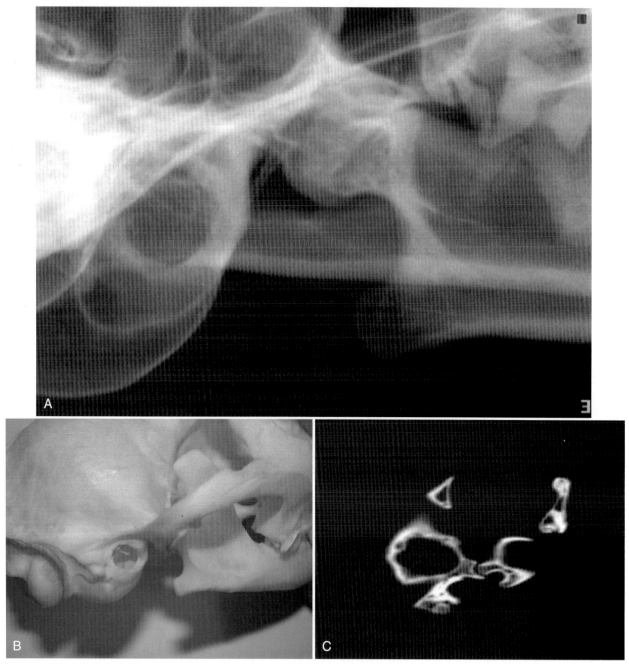

**FIGURE 4.6** Right temporomandibular joint (TMJ) in a cat. **A,** Radiograph of the right TMJ from a cat skull, lateral view. **B,** Lateral view of right TMJ from a prepared cat skull.

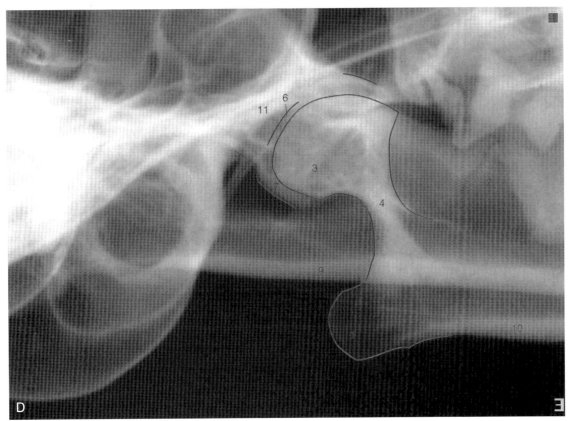

FIGURE 4.6, cont'd **C,** Transverse cut from a CT scan of a cat skull. **D,** Same radiograph as **A.**

1. Angular process of mandible (*os mandibulae, processus angularis*)
2. Body of the left mandible (*corpus mandibulae*)
3. Condylar process of mandible (*os mandibulae, processus condylaris, caput mandibulae*)
4. Neck of the condylar process of the mandible (*os mandibulae, processus condylaris, collum mandibulae*)
5. Mandibular canal (*canalis mandibulae*)
6. Mandibular fossa of temporal bone (*os temporal, fossa mandibularis*)
7. Retroarticular process of temporal bone (*os temporal, processus retroarticulatis*)
8. Tympanic bulla (*bulla tympanica*)
9. Ventral cortex of left mandible (*os mandibulae*)
10. Ventral cortex of the right mandible (*os mandibulae*)
11. Zygomatic process of temporal bone (*os temporal, processus zygomaticus*)

# CHAPTER 5

# Periodontal Disease

Dental radiographs assist in the assessment of periodontitis by providing information regarding alveolar bone loss. Dental radiographs are made to complement, not replace, the clinical examination. The clinical examination is essential for evaluating the soft tissue changes such as inflammation, gingival recession, and periodontal pocket formation (Figure 5-1). Clinical examination will provide evidence of mild bone loss, such as a Grade I furcation exposure, prior to changes being apparent on a dental radiograph. Dental probing as part of the clinical examination will detect vertical bone loss affecting the palatal aspect of the canine tooth, whereas it may not be detectable on a dental radiograph. This vertical bone loss may be associated with an unapparent oronasal fistula that can be identified on clinical but not radiographic examination. The dental radiograph is a two-dimensional image, and the morphology of an infrabony defect will be determined on clinical examination rather than on radiographic evaluation.

Dental radiographs are an important diagnostic tool when developing periodontal treatment plans. The extent and consequences (i.e., perio-endo lesion) of alveolar bone loss are determined from clinical and radiographic examination. Dental radiographs are also used as a means of monitoring disease progression and treatments.

Periodontitis is present when the alveolar bone has been affected, resulting in attachment loss. Radiographic evidence of periodontitis may be localized, affecting a single tooth or area of the mouth, or may be generalized, affecting multiple areas throughout the mouth. Widening of the periodontal ligament space, decreased alveolar bone density, and bone loss are all radiographic changes associated with periodontitis.

Terms used to describe the alveolar bone loss associated with periodontitis include:
- Alveolar margin bone loss
- Furcation bone loss
- Horizontal bone loss
- Vertical bone loss
- Combination of horizontal and vertical bone loss

Dental radiographs made for the evaluation of early alveolar bone loss should not be overexposed because this may result in "burn-out" of the alveolar marginal and interdental marginal bone. Dental radiographs should be made at the correct exposure or slightly under-exposed to provide the best detail when evaluating for early bone loss (Figure 5-2).

Alveolar bone loss may be mild, moderate, or severe, depending on the severity and chronicity of periodontitis (Figures 5-3, 5-4, and 5-5). In an individual patient, the significance of the bone loss will depend on the amount of attachment loss and the teeth involved. A toy or small-breed dog has much less alveolar bone than a larger-breed dog, and therefore an equal amount of alveolar bone loss will have more serious consequences for the smaller dogs compared to the larger dogs.

Furcation bone loss is bone loss that occurs in the area where multirooted teeth divide. It is assessed clinically by probing the furcation area with a dental explorer. Minimal furcation bone loss will not be detected radiographically. Approximately 30% to 40% of the furcation bone must be lost before it will be evident on a radiograph. A Grade 3 furcation exposure is complete loss of bone in the furcation area, and this may be identified readily on most two-rooted teeth but may be more difficult to determine on the three-rooted maxillary molar teeth (Figure 5-6).

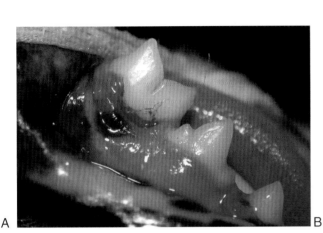
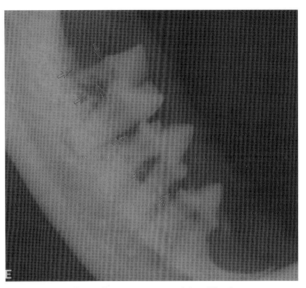

**FIGURE 5-1  A,** Photograph of a cat with inflamed gingiva and furcation exposure (identified on probing) of the right mandibular first molar. **B,** Severe alveolar bone loss (*open arrows*) and resorptive lesions (*arrows*) affecting the right mandibular first molar of the cat in **A.**

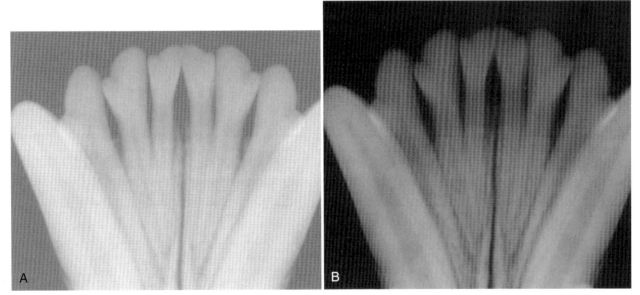

**FIGURE 5-2** Interdental alveolar marginal bone in a dog. **A,** The interdental and alveolar marginal bone is easier to visualize when the dental radiograph is underexposed. **B,** Overexposure results in burn-out of the interdental and alveolar marginal bone.

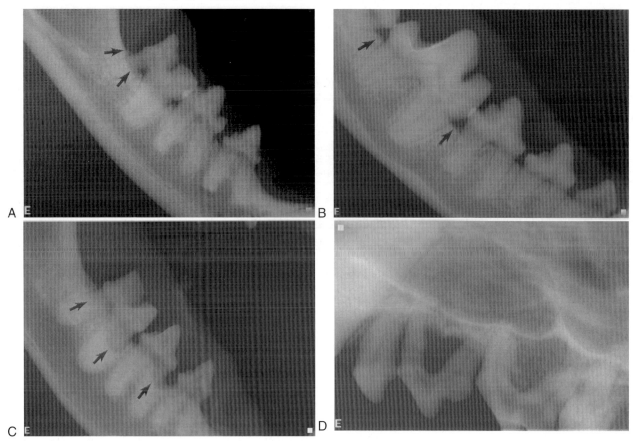

**FIGURE 5-3 Dental radiographs of patients with periodontitis. A,** Horizontal bone loss (*arrows*) around the distal root of the first molar in a cat. **B,** Horizontal bone loss (*arrows*) of the alveolar marginal bone on either side of the first molar in a dog. **C,** Alveolar bone loss (*arrows*) superimposed over the tooth roots in a cat. **D,** Severe horizontal bone loss in a dog.

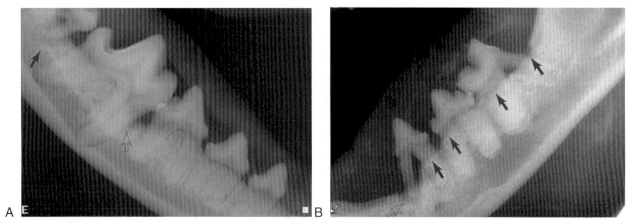

**FIGURE 5-4 A,** Vertical bone loss, moderate (*open arrow*) and severe (*arrow*) in a canine patient. **B,** Horizontal bone loss (*arrows*), furcation exposure, and severe vertical bone loss (*open arrow*) in a feline patient.

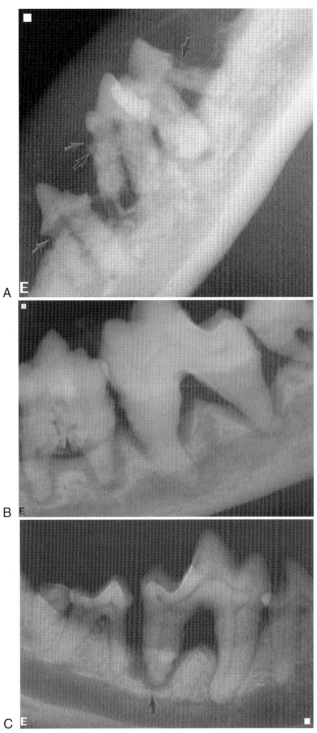

**FIGURE 5-5 A,** Partially luxated fourth premolar, severe alveolar bone loss, root resorption (arrows) and a rough appearance to the roots from calculus (*open arrow*) adhered to the tooth roots. **B,** Severe bone loss (furcation, horizontal and vertical) and calculus accumulation (*arrow*). **C,** Vertical bone loss extending around the entire distal root of the mandibular first molar (*arrow*).

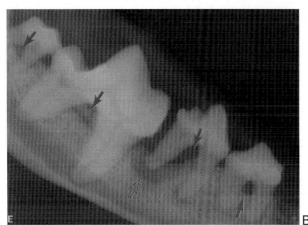

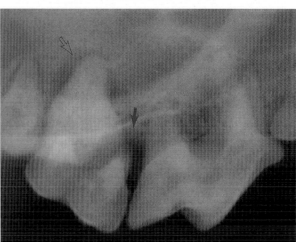

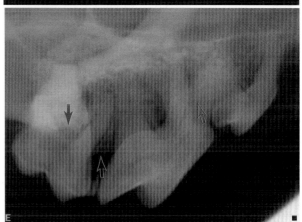

**FIGURE 5-6 A,** Furcation bone loss (*arrows*) of the mandibular third and fourth premolar and first and second molar. Vertical bone loss extending to the apex (*open arrow*) of the distal root of the fourth premolar. **B,** Decreased density of alveolar bone, from bone loss, in the furcation area between the mesial and distal roots of the fourth premolar. Complete attachment loss around the mesial-buccal root of the first molar (*arrow*) and a periapical lucency around the palatal root of the first molar (*open arrow*). **C,** A triangular lucency (*arrow*) is the result of furcation bone loss in the first molar. There is also furcation bone loss of the third and fourth premolar, and horizontal bone loss around the fourth premolar and first molar (*open arrows*).

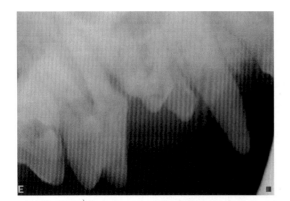

**FIGURE 5-7** Radiograph of a pug with crowding of teeth and a missing premolar. The first and second premolars are superimposed, making it difficult to evaluate the alveolar bone.

Crowded and malpositioned teeth make it more difficult to diagnose alveolar margin and furcation bone loss from a radiograph (Figure 5-7). Interdental alveolar bone loss and furcation bone loss, especially when mild, are often easier to identify radiographically than alveolar bone loss superimposed over the tooth roots (see Figure 5-3, *C*).

Severe periodontitis may result in secondary complications such as external root resorption and endodontic disease (Figure 5-8) or weakening of the mandible with potential for fracture (Figure 5-9).

Dental radiographs are necessary to evaluate treatment outcomes such as the success of guided tissue regeneration (GTR) (Figure 5-10).

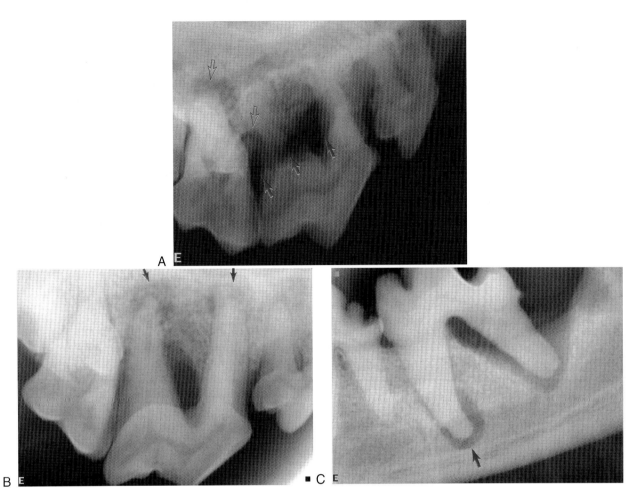

**FIGURE 5-8** Severe, chronic periodontitis may cause external root resorption or result in secondary endodontic disease. **A,** Generalized severe alveolar bone loss, external root resorption (*arrows*) on the fourth premolar, and periapical bone loss around the first molar (*open arrows*). **B,** Severe bone loss in the furcation area and periapical lucencies (*arrows*) consistent with chronic endodontic disease of the fourth premolar. **C,** Severe horizontal and vertical bone loss extending to the apex of the distal root of the first molar. The periapical lucency (*arrow*) of the mesial root is compatible with endodontic disease. The severe periodontitis of the distal root may have lead to the endodontic disease.

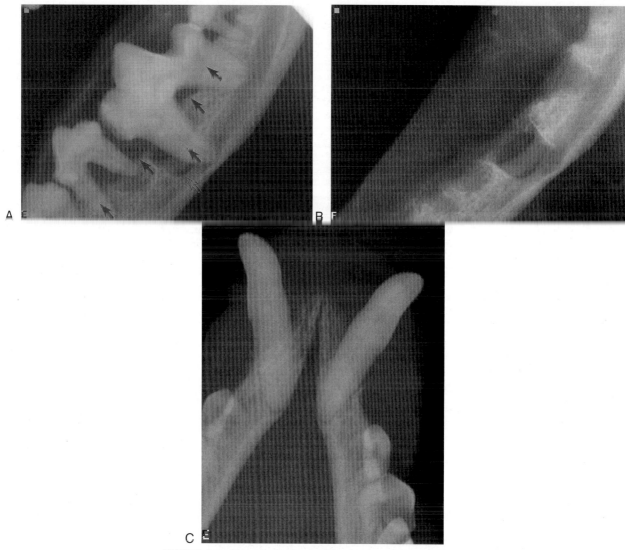

**FIGURE 5-9** Chronic periodontitis can result in sufficient bone loss to increase the risk of fracture during an extraction, when chewing on hard foods, toys, or treats or with minor trauma. **A,** Dental radiograph from a small breed dog with chronic, severe periodontitis. The severe alveolar bone loss as demonstrated by the furcation exposure, horizontal bone loss (*arrows*), and vertical bone loss (*open arrow*) place the mandible at an increased risk for fracture. **B,** Radiograph from same dog in **A** after the extractions have been completed. **C,** Chronic periodontitis has resulted in loss of the mandibular incisors, the associated alveolar bone and severe bone loss around the canines.

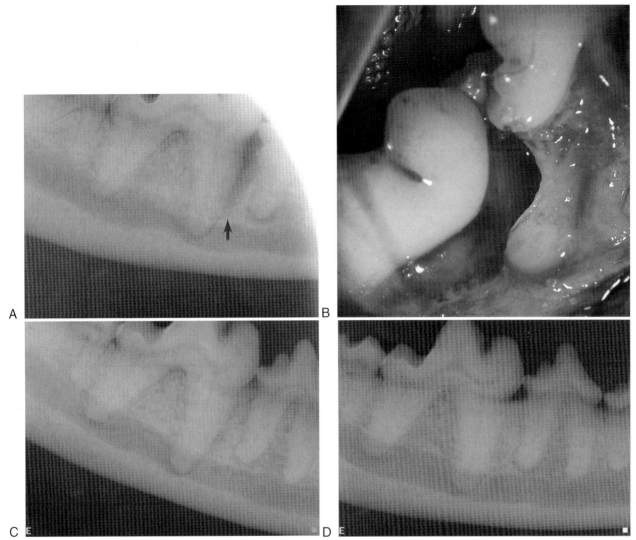

**FIGURE 5-10** Clinical photograph and dental radiographs from a dog that had an infrabony pocket treated with guided tissue regeneration (GTR). **A,** The initial radiograph made to evaluate the bone loss identified on periodontal probing. On the radiograph there is severe vertical bone loss on the mesial aspect of the mesial root of the right lower first molar (*arrow*). **B,** Photograph of the infrabony pocket after the soft tissue has been removed. Surgical exposure revealed the morphology of the infrabony pocket better than the dental radiograph. **C,** Dental radiograph made immediately after the GTR procedure was completed. On the radiograph there is filling of the infrabony defect with the radiodense material used for the procedure. **D,** Radiograph of patient in **A, B,** and **C,** taken 2 years later. The radiograph is characterized by a normal alveolar margin height around the right lower first molar.

# CHAPTER 6

# Endodontic Disease

Radiography is a vital component of veterinary endodontic treatment. Radiographs provide information about the presence, nature, and severity of periapical and root pathology. This information is essential for the diagnosis of endodontic disease as well as for the prognosis of its treatment. Radiographs do not provide direct information about pulp health; however, many of the effects of pulp pathology are radiographically visible.

Clinical findings that may indicate the presence of endodontic disease include a fractured tooth with exposure of the pulp chamber, a discolored tooth, or an intraoral or extraoral draining fistula. Except in the obvious case of a direct pulp exposure, a definitive diagnosis of endodontic pathology is difficult to make based only on clinical examination of veterinary patients due to the limitations of pulp testing and lack of patient input. Also, endodontic disease can be present with very little clinical evidence. This is particularly true of maxillary molar teeth that can develop severe periodontitis with extension to the endodontic tissues while exhibiting no clinical signs other than slight mobility (Figure 6-1).

Human patients with endodontic pathology experience various symptoms that range from very mild discomfort when the tooth is loaded in the presence of apical periodontitis, to severe persistent pain when there is an acute apical abscess. These symptoms alert human patients to the existence of a problem, which they can communicate to a dentist. In contrast, veterinary patients often tolerate significant discomfort without complaint. We are forced to rely on radiographic evidence of endodontic disease (Figure 6-2). Radiographs should be made of teeth that are fractured, close to a draining fistula, intrinsically discolored, anomalous, or compromised from periodontal disease to determine the extent of the problem and to evaluate the endodontic and periradicular health.

Dental radiographs can be misleading and unreliable. Early endodontic disease may not show any radiographic abnormalities, while superimposed anatomy can mimic

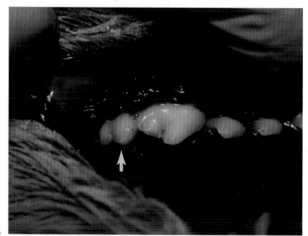

A

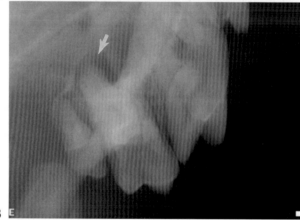

B

**FIGURE 6-1 A,** The first molar tooth (*arrow*) and adjacent periodontal tissues appear relatively normal. **B,** The palatal root is characterized by periradicular bone loss and a large area of periapical lucency (*arrow*).

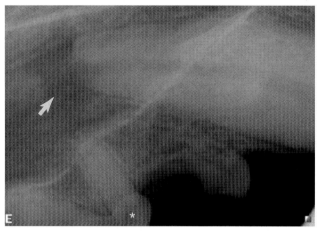

**FIGURE 6-2** The second premolar tooth appears radiographically normal, but the canine tooth has an endodontic lesion (*arrow*). An incidental finding is an anomalous and resorbing first premolar tooth. This patient's only clinical symptom was a draining fistula adjacent to the left maxillary second premolar tooth (*asterisk*).

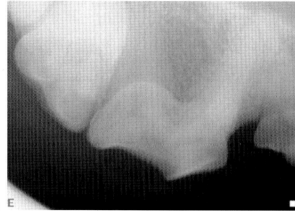

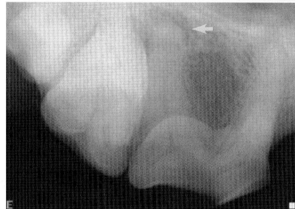

**FIGURE 6-3 A,** A radiograph of a right maxillary fourth premolar tooth that has a crown fracture. The visible root apices appear normal. **B,** On a correctly positioned radiograph, a periapical lucency of endodontic origin is evident on the distal root (*arrow*).

endodontic disease on a radiograph of a healthy tooth. Despite these limitations, dental radiographs continue to be the best tool available to evaluate endodontic health in veterinary patients. It is important for veterinarians to become familiar with radiographic assessment of periapical tissues. In humans, it has been determined that both the accuracy of diagnostic decisions and the probability of appropriate treatment decisions increased when a dentist was confident about his or her diagnosis or treatment. It seems likely that this also holds true for veterinarians practicing dentistry. The more confidence we have in our radiographic diagnosis of pathology, the better and more efficient will be the treatment we provide for our patients.

## Radiographic Signs of Endodontic Disease

Inflammation caused by endodontic disease affects the surrounding bone and teeth, resulting in changes that can be radiographically detected. Radiographs that are meant to evaluate the periapical tissues should include the entire root tip and surrounding bone (Figure 6-3). They should also be well positioned to avoid elongation, foreshortening, angulation, or distortion of the image. The compact bone that forms the walls of the alveolus (the white line of the lamina dura on radiographs) is also referred to as a cribriform plate due to its multiple perforations for vessels and nerves. This bone is very sensitive to inflammatory mediators that originate in the pulp and escape into the surrounding periodontal ligament. The bone responds with osteoclastic resorption. The characteristic radiographic lesion of endodontic origin (LEO) involves changes in the periapical radiodensity or detail that result from apical periodontitis. LEOs can also develop along

the lateral aspect of a root at the site of a lateral canal. Other radiographic signs of endodontic disease are caused by the effects of inflammation or pulp death on the tooth itself.

Radiographic signs of endodontic disease that are associated with the tissues around tooth roots include:
- Increased width of the apical radiolucent periodontal ligament space
- Loss of the radiopaque lamina dura at the apex or other portals of exit such as lateral canals
- Diffuse periapical radiolucency with indistinct borders that may indicate an acute abscess
- Clearly evident periapical radiolucency with distinct borders that is evidence of a more chronic lesion
- Diffuse area of radiopacity where low-grade chronic inflammation results in sclerosing osteitis
- Changes in the trabecular bone pattern around the root apex

Radiographic signs of endodontic disease that are associated with the tooth itself include:
- Root tip resorption
- Internal root or crown resorption

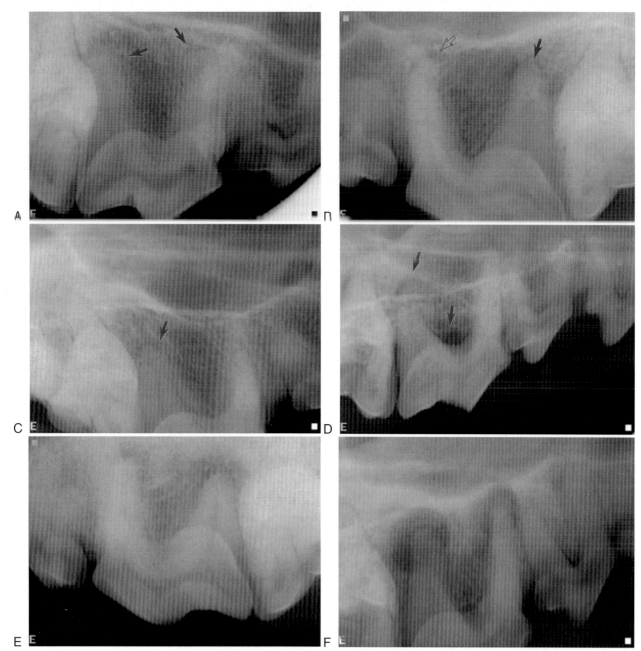

**FIGURE 6-4 Lesions of endodontic origin. A,** The periodontal ligament at the apex of the distal and mesiobuccal roots is wider than normal (*arrows*). This is one of the earliest radiographic signs of apical periodontitis. **B,** The distal root has lost the lamina dura in an area of irregular radiolucency (*arrow*). The mesiobuccal root has a more extensive loss of the lamina dura (*open arrow*). **C,** External resorption of the distal root tip created an irregular defect (*arrow*). **D,** The lamina dura is clearly absent over a larger area of the distal root and in the furcation area (*arrows*). **E,** The mesiobuccal and distal roots have diffuse periapical radiolucencies with indistinct borders. This is typical of an acute apical abscess. **F,** Large radiolucencies with very distinct borders are typical of chronic apical periodontitis. This is consistent with a cyst or a granuloma.

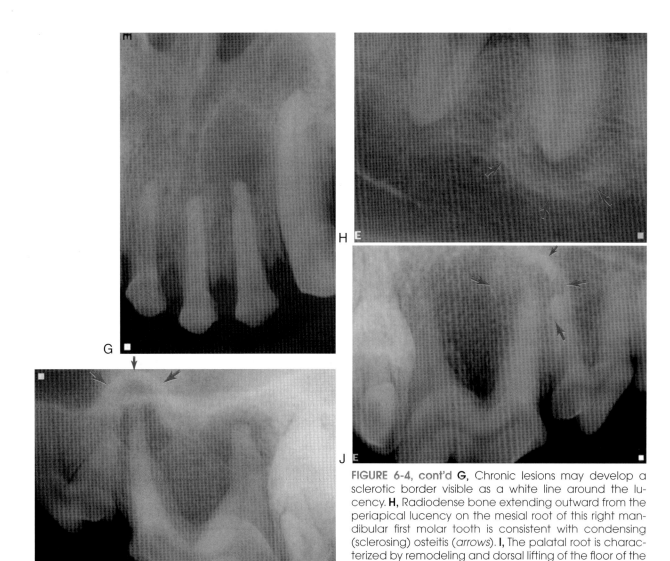

FIGURE 6-4, cont'd **G,** Chronic lesions may develop a sclerotic border visible as a white line around the lucency. **H,** Radiodense bone extending outward from the periapical lucency on the mesial root of this right mandibular first molar tooth is consistent with condensing (sclerosing) osteitis (*arrows*). **I,** The palatal root is characterized by remodeling and dorsal lifting of the floor of the nasal cavity just rostral to the maxillary recess (*arrows*). In humans with lifting of the sinus floor this radiographic finding has been called the "halo effect." **J,** One of the mesial roots shows periapical condensing osteitis without an associated lucency (*arrows*). There is increased radiopacity and loss of the trabecular bone pattern.

- External root resorption (distinct from the dental tooth resorption of idiopathic origin, see Chapter 7)
- Arrested tooth maturation (pulp necrosis)
- Accelerated apparent tooth maturation (pulpitis)

A necrotic or severely inflamed pulp produces inflammatory mediators that can exit the tooth through the apical delta and lateral canals, stimulating leukocyte infiltration and edema. Inflammatory bone resorption at these sites form radiographic LEOs. The earliest extracanal inflammation to occur is usually acute apical periodontitis. Radiographically, this either appears as widening of the apical periodontal ligament space or as no change at all (Figure 6-4, *A*). Bone and root resorption occur at this stage but the changes may be too small to appear radio-

graphically; lack of a radiographic lesion does not rule out early endodontic disease. Another early radiographic sign is loss of the apical lamina dura (Figure 6-4, *B–D*). This is also not a reliable indicator of disease because the apical lamina dura frequently becomes unidentifiable when there is insufficient overlying radiodense tissue. Humans report sensitivity to percussion at this early stage when radiographic changes are difficult to identify.

Another acute form of disease is an acute apical abscess caused by severe inflammation from a necrotic pulp. Radiographically, this can range from increased width of the periodontal ligament space to a large region of mild-to-moderate periapical lucency with indistinct borders (Figure 6-4, *E*). When an abscess subsides, much of the demineralized bone can remineralize, resulting in a smaller radiolucency that has more definite borders.

Chronic apical periodontitis usually results in formation of a cyst or granuloma that appears radiographically as an obvious radiolucency with distinct borders (Figure 6-4, *F, G*). This can be associated with minimal symptoms in humans. The border of the cyst or granuloma can also show evidence of increased radiopacity due to sclerosing osteitis or focal sclerosing osteomyelitis (Figure 6-4, *H*). When this expands the alveolar bone into the nasal cavity, it can appear radiographically similar to the "antral halo" described in humans. The palatal root of the maxillary fourth premolar tooth in dogs can create a similar halo effect where the expanding bone protrudes upward into the nasal cavity (Figure 6-4, *I*). Another form of chronic apical periodontitis is condensing, or sclerosing, osteitis that appears as a diffuse increase in radiodensity with or without a radiolucency (Figure 6-4, *J*).

Although the features of a radiographic lucency can suggest the nature of the apical lesion, they cannot reliably distinguish between an apical cyst, granuloma, or abscess. Extracted teeth that are endodontically affected frequently have granulomatous tissue attached to the root tips (Figure 6-5). Apical inflammation can progress to suppurative apical periodontitis. When this occurs, the inflammation and suppuration can dissect through tissues (Figure 6-6) to form a draining fistula. Fistulas from endodontically involved maxillary incisor and canine teeth commonly exit at the mucogingival line (MGL) directly below the root apex, while fistulas from affected premolar teeth commonly appear at the MGL in the furcation area. This is because the inflammatory process dissects through tissues following the path of least resistance. After traveling under the loosely attached alveolar mucosa, it encounters the firmly attached gingiva where it deviates to the surface at the mucogingival line. The mesiobuccal and distal roots of the maxillary fourth premolar tooth often drain externally on the skin of the face below the eye, where it can be misdiagnosed as a primary skin problem unrelated to the teeth. Mandibular canine teeth commonly drain in the vestibular mucosa or skin of the ventral mandible, and mandibular first molar teeth commonly drain intraorally in the interradicular area but can also dissect to more remote locations. The site of exit does not always directly correlate to the problem tooth. Radiographs are needed to determine which tooth is involved (Figure 6-7).

In addition to periapical and periradicular (lateral canal) LEOs, other radiographic signs of endodontic pathology are associated with the teeth themselves. Inflammation in the periodontal ligament can cause external root resorption, while inflammation of the pulp can cause internal resorption (Figures 6-8 through 6-10). External resorption of the root tip can complicate achieving an apical seal during endodontic treatment, while internal resorption can make it more challenging to get a three-dimensional canal preparation and

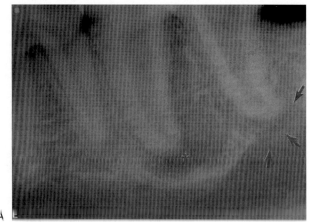

A

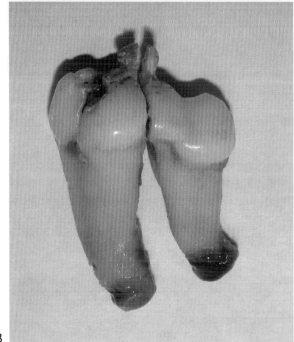

B

**FIGURE 6-5 A,** Both roots of a left mandibular first molar tooth have periapical lucencies. The lesion on the mesial root has a very clear lucency surrounded by an encircling opacity (*asterisk*). This radiographic appearance has been classically considered to indicate a cyst or granuloma. The radiographic lesion on the distal root (*arrows*) has less distinct borders and the lucency is less pronounced. These findings have been described as characteristic of an apical abscess. However, the nature of the apical pathology cannot be reliably determined radiographically. **B,** Both of the extracted root tips have granulomatous tissue attached to the apices. The radiographs may commonly overestimate the size of the apical granuloma or cyst. This tooth has a deformed crown caused by previous trauma to the developing tooth bud as a puppy.

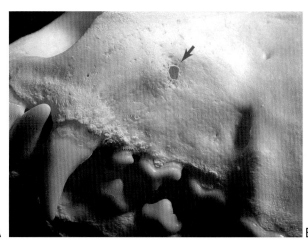 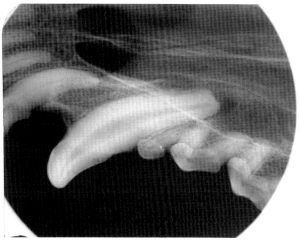

A B

**FIGURE 6-6 A,** Skull with fenestration (*arrow*) of the buccal bone over the root apex caused by an untreated endodontic problem. The tooth appeared normal except for slight crown discoloration. **B,** On a radiograph of the skull, the canine tooth has a periapical lucency typical of LEOs. The radiolucency has a rounded apex, unlike the tapered apex of a normal chevron lucency. Also note that the root canal and pulp chamber are larger than expected compared to the adjacent teeth.

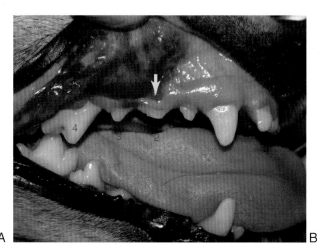 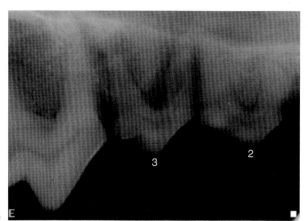

A B

**FIGURE 6-7 A,** A right maxillary second premolar tooth has abrasional crown wear and a draining fistula between its roots (*arrow*). **B,** Radiograph of the patient in **A.** The second premolar tooth shown in **A** appears radiographically normal, but the third premolar tooth has periodontal disease, endodontic disease, and external root resorption. Surgery confirmed the infection had dissected from the third premolar tooth around the distal root of the second premolar to the furcation area. The second, third, and fourth premolar teeth are labeled 2, 3, and 4, respectively.

*Continued.*

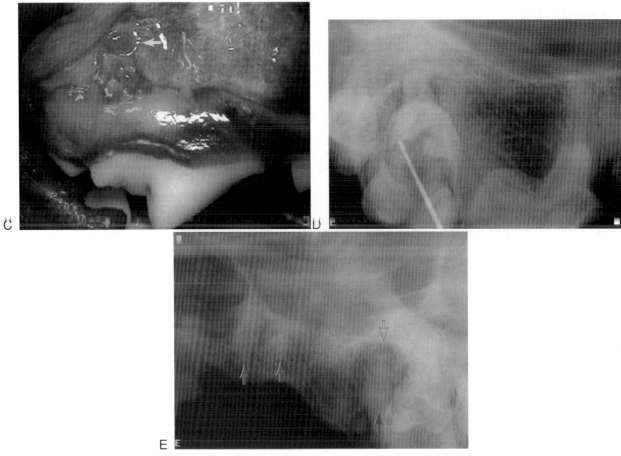

FIGURE 6-7, cont'd C, A parulis marks a draining tract adjacent to the distal root of the right maxillary fourth premolar tooth (*arrow*). D, A gutta percha point in the fistulous tract traces the source of the infection to the first molar tooth. The fourth premolar is undergoing resorption. The radiograph is taken from a more dorsal angle than the photograph, which projects the fistula opening more ventral (coronal) on the radiograph. E, This patient had the left maxillary fourth premolar tooth extracted, and the associated facial fistula surgically closed 6 months previously. Continued facial drainage was caused by persistent infected roots (*arrows*). There is a periapical lucency around the distal root (*open arrow*).

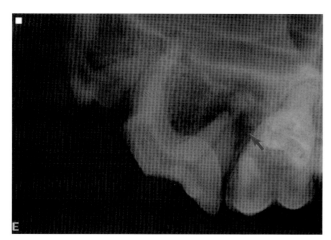

FIGURE 6-8 External root resorption (*arrow*) affecting the distal root of a left maxillary fourth premolar tooth. The pulp chamber was exposed at the middle pulp horn from an open fracture.

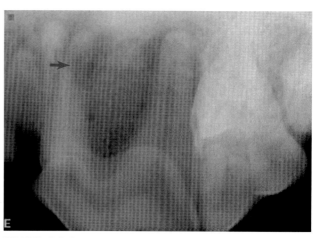

FIGURE 6-9 The mesiobuccal root of the left maxillary fourth premolar tooth has an area of internal and external root resorption (*arrow*). There are radiolucent areas around all three root tips.

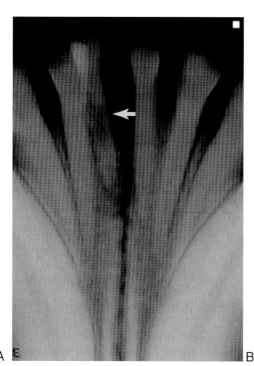

A

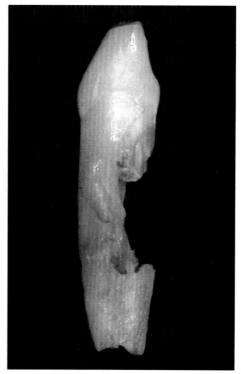

B

FIGURE 6-10 **A,** The right mandibular first incisor tooth has a mid-root radiolucency (*arrow*) that could be either internal resorption (widened canal) or external resorption on the mid-facial or mid-lingual surface. There is also periapical lucency, supereruption (it appears to be exfoliating), and tipping of the tooth. **B,** Side view of the extracted tooth. The damage affected the entire mid-lingual region of the root from the periodontal ligament to the root canal.

internal fill (Figure 6-11). Dental radiographs do not always fully reflect the extent of resorptive damage to the root (Figure 6-12). In contrast to internal resorption that removes dentin from the wall of the pulp cavity, pulpitis can also result in formation of tertiary, or reparative, dentin on the walls of the pulp cavity. Pulpitis that is generalized over a section of a root canal creates the radiographic effect of a narrower canal in that section, giving the appearance of a more mature tooth. The extreme of this can manifest as "pulp cavity obliteration," a radiographic term that describes an inability to identify sections of, or the entire, pulp space (Figure 6-13). The term "pulp canal obliteration" is most commonly used to describe an abnormal rather than a physiological pulp chamber and root canal deposition of mineral-dense material. The calcific metamorphosis of advanced age has a similar radiographic appearance to accelerated dentin production. Whether due to advanced age or to trauma to the pulp or its vascular supply, the root canal still physically exists, although it can be very attenuated. Pulp necrosis causes the opposite effect, arresting any further dentin formation or tooth maturation. The result is a tooth that appears radiographically less mature (wider root canal space) than the adjacent teeth (Figure 6-14). Endodontic lesions in cats appear radiographically similar to those in dogs (Figure 6-15).

## Lucencies That Can Mimic Endodontic Lesions

Apical radiographs can be challenging to interpret due to the two-dimensional depiction of complicated anatomy that combines trabecular (spongy) bone, compact bone, soft tissue, and air spaces all projected at various angles and configurations. A radiolucency that commonly mimics an LEO is the "chevron lucency" that can be associated with the root apices of incisor and canine teeth (see Chapter 2). It is differentiated from a true endodontic lesion by its regular chevron shape compared with the more circular or irregular-shaped lucencies often seen in LEOs. Other confusing lucencies and opacities can be created by the summation effect of superimposed structures, projecting overlying anatomy in a way that makes it appear to be associated with a tooth root or its supporting bone. These can include bony foramena, bony fissures, bony canals, and trabeculae. Many nonpathological lucencies, opacities, and apparent deviations from normal can be distinguished from true lesions by comparison with a radiograph of the contralateral tooth.

## Etiology

Two categories of insult that most commonly cause endodontic disease are bacterial infection and dental trauma. Dental pulp responds to injury in a manner similar to that of other connective tissues. However, the circulation is very limited and the tissue is confined within a rigid space that restricts

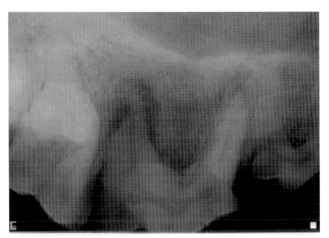

FIGURE 6-11 The large external resorption on the distal root of the right maxillary fourth premolar tooth makes it a poor candidate for conventional endodontic therapy.

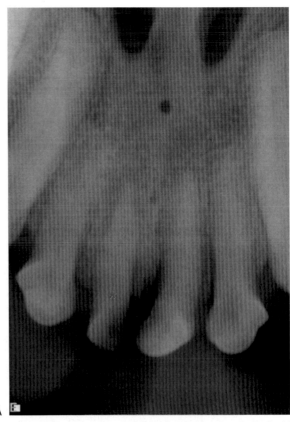

FIGURE 6-12 **A,** The right maxillary first incisor tooth (*asterisk*) has a shortened root tip with a narrow apex.

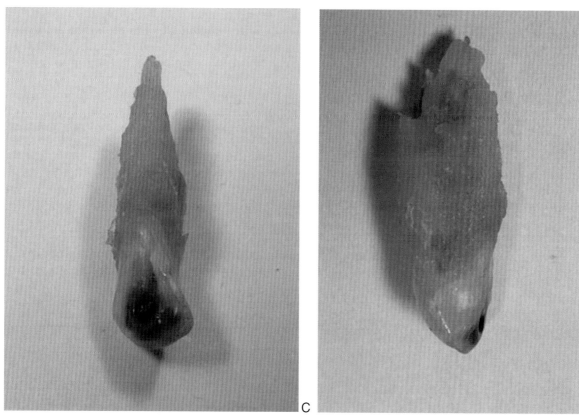

B                                          C

**FIGURE 6-12, cont'd B,** In the buccolingual view the extracted tooth appears as depicted in the radiograph. **C,** In side view (mesiodistal dimension), a view not available to dental radiography in a patient, the extent of the damage is visible.

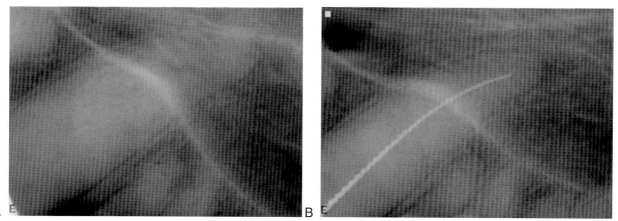

A                                          B

**FIGURE 6-13 A,** The root canal is difficult to visualize in this left maxillary canine tooth. This is common in very mature teeth or in cases of chronic pulpitis. **B,** The endodontic file demonstrates that the root canal is still present, even though radiographically unapparent.

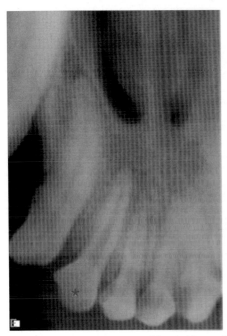

FIGURE 6-14 The root canal space of the right maxillary second incisor tooth (*asterisk*) is wider than those of the other incisors, indicating pulp necrosis and arrested maturation.

its ability to swell. Trauma, inflammation, or infection of the pulp tissue can either heal or progress to irreversible pulpitis or pulp necrosis.

When the pulp of a mature tooth is exposed to the oral cavity, the pulp will eventually become infected and irreversibly inflamed, generally leading to pulp necrosis. A fractured or worn tooth that has a direct exposure of the pulp chamber requires root canal treatment or extraction (Figure 6-16). In very specific cases, a vital direct pulp cap procedure may be done. But an exposed pulp will not heal without intervention. A client should never be advised to "watch it to see if it develops a problem."

Bacteria can also enter the endodontic system of a non-traumatized tooth through extension of periodontal disease. If the periodontal epithelial attachment migrates apically to an endodontic vascular entrance such as a lateral canal, furcation communication, or the apical foramen or delta, then the pulp could become infected (Figure 6-17). This is referred to as a primary periodontal lesion with secondary endodontic involvement (it has also been referred to as a "perio-endo lesion"). These most commonly occur in patients suffering from generalized periodontitis, but they can also occur from localized secondary periodontal disease

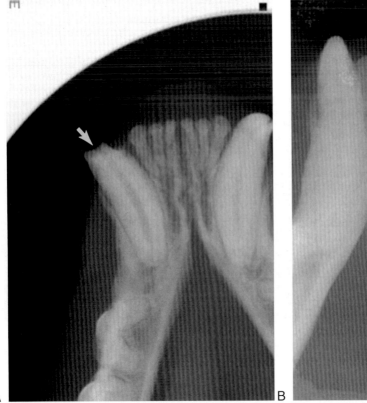

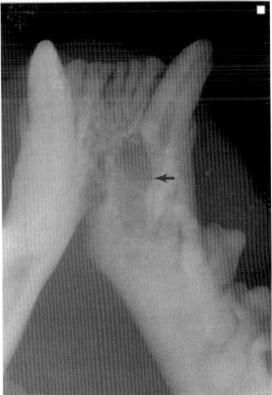

A          B

FIGURE 6-15 Radiographic signs of endodontic disease are similar in cats. **A,** The right mandibular canine tooth (*arrow*) has a fractured crown, a wider pulp than the left, and periapical lucency. **B,** The left mandibular canine tooth in this cat is characterized by the same three abnormalities as the patient in **A,** plus extensive external root resorption (*arrow*).

such as that caused by periodontal foreign bodies or transpalatal objects wedged between the upper fourth premolar teeth (Figure 6-18). Apical and radicular LEOs can dissect coronally along the side of the root to exit in the sulcus, creating a primary endodontic lesion with secondary periodontal disease (has also been referred to as an "endo-perio lesion"). The bony defects around a tooth with primary endodontic disease and concurrent but unrelated periodontal disease can meet to form a combined periodontal and endodontic lesion (Figure 6-19).

Pulp inflammation and necrosis can also result from deep dental caries with extension of the bacterial infection to the pulp (see Chapter 11).

Blunt trauma can cause pulp hemorrhage and endodontic disease even when the tooth crown does not fracture. The breakdown products of extravasated blood in the dentinal tubules discolor the tooth pink immediately after the injury. Over time, the tooth becomes darker brown or gray

and the crown is less able to transilluminate light. Although the pulp has some ability to heal after mild trauma, the most common result of pulp trauma is irreversible pulpitis even when there is no bacterial contamination of the pulp (see Figure 6-6). Radiographic signs depend on the pulp response (Figures 6-20 and 6-21).

## Endodontic Treatment

Preprocedural radiographs help to determine whether a tooth is a good candidate for endodontic treatment. They also provide information about the root canal morphology (Figures 6-22 and 6-23).

During the endodontic procedure, radiographs should be made to determine the working length of the root canal and to identify problems such as extension of obturating materials beyond the root apex, filling short of the root canal terminus, poor adaptation of the fill to the root canal walls,

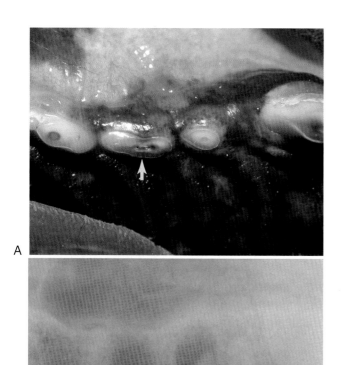

A

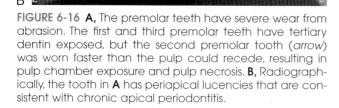

B

FIGURE 6-16 **A,** The premolar teeth have severe wear from abrasion. The first and third premolar teeth have tertiary dentin exposed, but the second premolar tooth (*arrow*) was worn faster than the pulp could recede, resulting in pulp chamber exposure and pulp necrosis. **B,** Radiographically, the tooth in **A** has periapical lucencies that are consistent with chronic apical periodontitis.

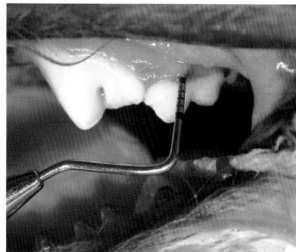

A

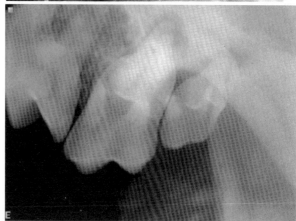

B

FIGURE 6-17 **Primary periodontal disease with secondary endodontic involvement. A,** A periodontal probe measures a 9-mm periodontal pocket on the buccal (vestibular) side of a left maxillary first molar tooth that appears clinically normal. **B,** All six roots of the molar teeth of the patient in **A** are characterized by loss of supportive bone and periapical lucency.

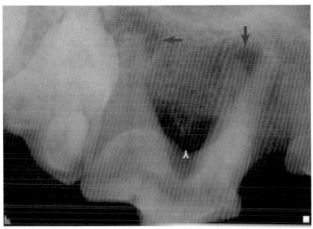

FIGURE 6-18 The right maxillary fourth premolar tooth appeared clinically normal except for palatal recession where a stick had been wedged across the palate between the fourth premolar teeth. Pressure necrosis was followed by infection in the furcation area that spread to the pulp. The lucency in the furcation area (*asterisk*) was the primary lesion, and the periapical lucencies (*arrows*) were secondary to endodontic extension.

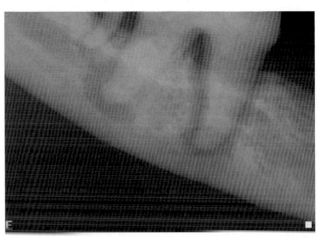

FIGURE 6-19 Combined periodontal and endodontic lesion. The right mandibular first molar tooth had dental caries and periodontal disease. On the radiograph, there is evidence of horizontal, oblique, and vertical bone loss from periodontitis and periapical lucency from concurrent endodontic disease.

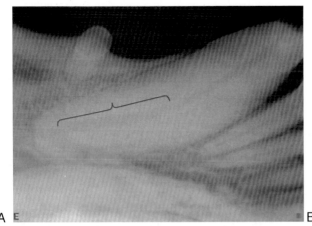

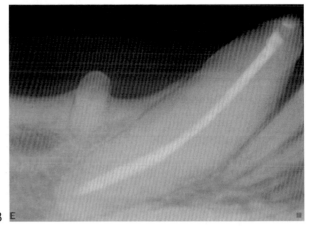

A

B

FIGURE 6-20 **A,** The right mandibular canine tooth was weakened and eventually fractured due to chronic fence biting. The pulp chamber and coronal half of the root canal are very narrow due to accelerated generalized tertiary, or reparative, dentin deposition from chronic pulpitis. The apical half of the root canal (*bracket*) is wider because it matured at a normal slower rate. **B,** Radiodense obturating material enhances visualization of the canal widths.

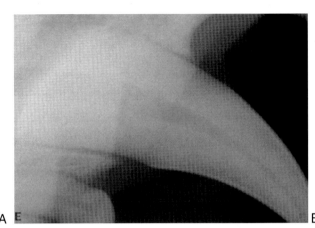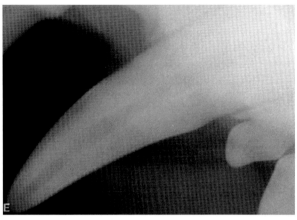

A E

B E

FIGURE 6-21 **A,** The pulp chamber of a canine tooth should have an even contour that matches the tooth surface contour. **B,** The contralateral tooth of the same patient as in **A** was discolored from previous pulp hemorrhage. While the root canal space is narrower than the normal tooth due to pulpitis similar to the tooth in Figure 6-20, the pulp chamber is wider than the pulp chamber in the normal tooth in **A** due to pulp necrosis and arrested maturation.

and voids in the fill or poor fill density (Figures 6-24 through 6-27).

Procedural radiographs also help to identify complications. During filing and canal preparation, the prepared canal can be redirected or iatrogenically transported from the original canal position. This can occur by ledging (Figure 6-28) when large files fail to navigate a curve, apical transportation when larger and stiffer files are instrumented to apical length, apical widening or elbowing, or strip perforation coronally on the inside curve and apically on the outside curve of a root. Timely radiographs identify these developing problems and facilitate their correction. Another complication that can occur during lateral compaction ("condensation") is vertical root fracture. Roots with one narrow dimension (for example, incisor teeth with a narrow mesiodistal dimension) are more at risk for this. Roots that split during compaction with a spreader can produce a soft cracking sound. Radiographically, this appears as a radiopaque line parallel to the wall of the root canal (Figure 6-29). Vertical root fractures are particularly difficult to identify and may not appear on a radiograph if the plane of the fracture is superimposed over the obturating material in the root canal. In humans, these cause pain when chewing or when horizontal force is applied to the tooth.

A postoperative radiograph should be made to evaluate the quality of the apical fill. The apex of normal mature dogs and cats has an apical delta with many small canaliculi (Figure 6-30). When these are not occluded with tissue or debris, some radiopaque sealant material can be extruded through the canaliculi to create an apical blush. The endodontic anatomy sometimes becomes apparent only after it has been three-dimensionally filled with radiopaque obturating material (Figure 6-31).

Feline endodontic radiography is similar to that in dogs. The most common teeth treated in cats are the canine teeth. Chronic endodontic inflammation in cats seems to result in

a higher incidence of root tip resorption and damage that can complicate root canal treatment (Figures 6-32 and 6-33).

The success of endodontic treatment is evaluated by making follow-up radiographs. Radiographic changes in the periapical bone can occur slowly (Figure 6-34). Follow-up radiographs are often taken 1 year postoperatively, and then again in 2 to 4 years. Unlike the dental pulp, the apical periodontal ligament has a rich blood supply that provides an excellent ability to heal. When the inciting cause of inflammation is removed, the inflammatory response decreases and tissue-forming cells increase, followed by tissue organization and maturation. The periodontal ligament, which is the first tissue to be damaged by the inflammation, is the last tissue to repair (Figure 6-35). Follow-up is even more important for cases that carry a more guarded prognosis due to materials outside the root canal space, procedural misadventures, anatomical challenges, or the possibility of difficult-to-resolve infection in the periapical tissues of chronic cases (Figure 6-36).

Follow-up radiographs that indicate failure often identify the cause of the failure (Figure 6-37). Correction of the problem and retreatment with conventional endodontic treatment is indicated. Sometimes the reason for failure is not obvious (Figure 6-38). Retreatment with conventional endodontic treatment can be performed, but it is also possible that a surgical approach to debride the periapical tissues and to place a root tip filling may be necessary in addition to conventional retreatment.

Pulp necrosis in an immature tooth results in periapical inflammation that arrests maturation of the apex. The apex remains open and does not form a delta. Procedures to resolve the inflammation and allow healing and apical closure (apexification or apexogenesis) require radiographic confirmation of success prior to definitive endodontic treatment (Figure 6-39).

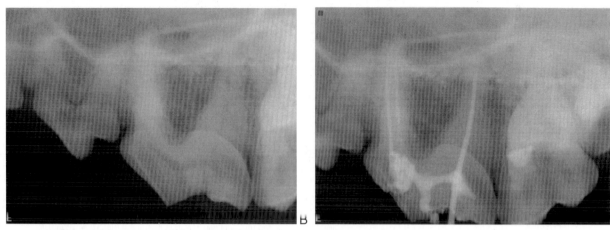

FIGURE 6-22 **A,** On a preprocedural radiograph, the narrow mesiobuccal and palatal root canals are difficult to discern. **B,** On an intraoperative radiograph, the canals have all been identified and treated.

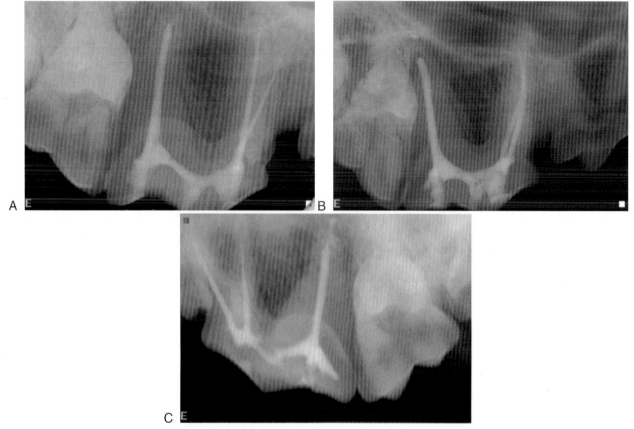

FIGURE 6-23 Variable root anatomy of the maxillary fourth premolar tooth. **A,** Relatively straight roots. **B,** Gently curved mesiobuccal and palatal roots. **C,** Divergent mesiobuccal and palatal roots.

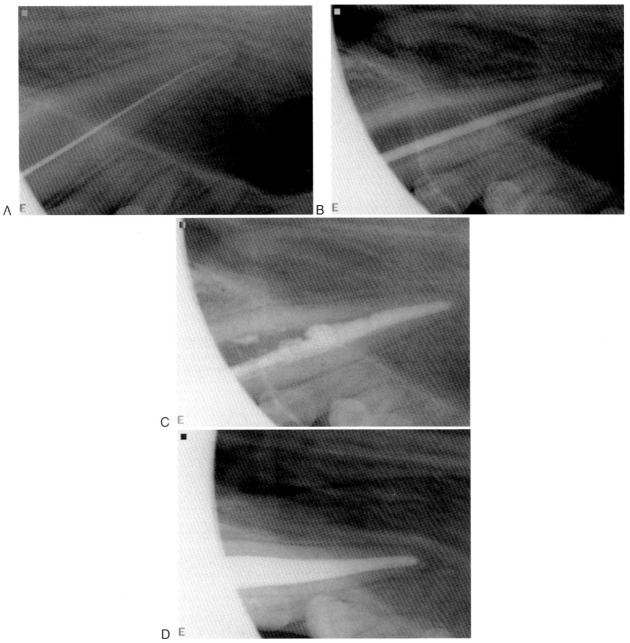

**FIGURE 6-24** Procedural radiographs during root canal treatment. **A,** Working length radiograph to confirm the distance to the root canal terminus. **B,** Master cone in place. **C,** Apical compaction and backfill. **D,** Postoperative.

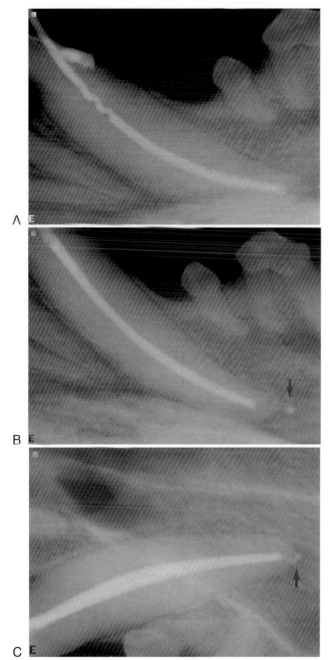

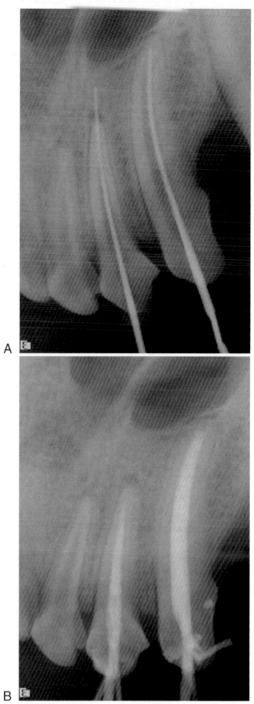

**FIGURE 6-25 A,** Long, narrow canal early in compaction procedure. **B,** As obturation progresses, sealant is forced through the canaliculi of the apical delta (arrows). **C,** Another obturation showing a "sealant blush" of extruded sealant (arrow). Small amounts of sealant like these would be expected to resorb over time. This is evidence that the apical delta is not blocked by necrotic tissue or debris.

**FIGURE 6-26 A,** On the procedural radiograph, the endodontic file passes through the apex of the second incisor tooth and into the periapical tissues. This establishes the presence of an open apical foramen instead of an apical delta. **B,** An apical stop has been recreated with endodontic files enabling materials to remain confined to the root canal space.

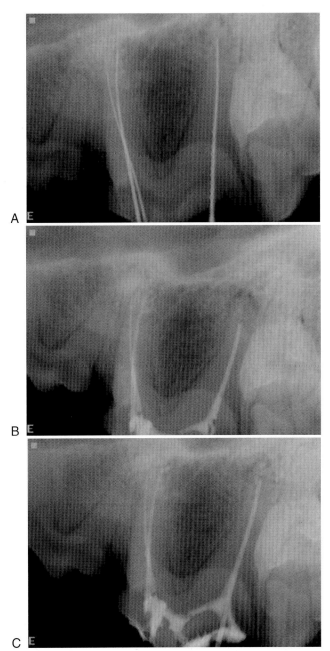

**FIGURE 6-27 A,** Files in the root canals confirm working lengths. **B,** The distal root is filled short of the canal terminus. **C,** The problem has been corrected.

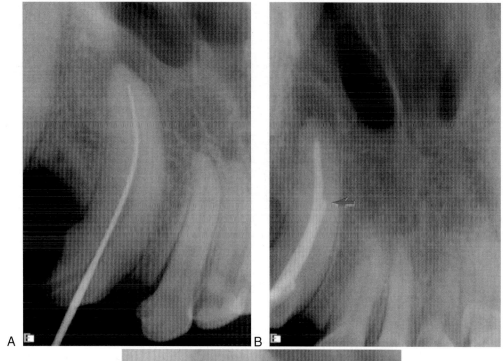

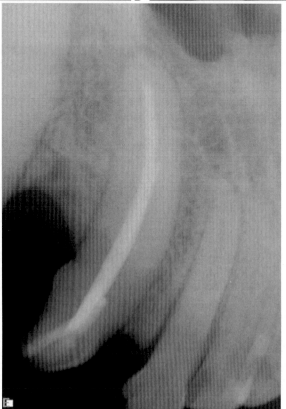

FIGURE 6-28 **A,** Curve in the root canal of a right maxillary third incisor tooth is predisposed to ledging. **B,** A ledge was made at the curve (*arrow*) followed by instrumentation and treatment past the ledge. **C,** On the 2-year follow-up radiograph, there is evidence of healing of the periapical defect.

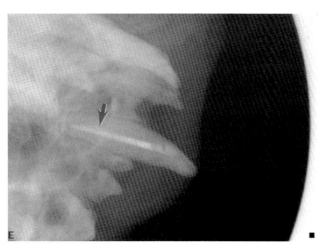

**FIGURE 6-29** Vertical root fracture appears as a radiopaque line parallel to the root canal (*arrow*). This carries a poor long-term prognosis.

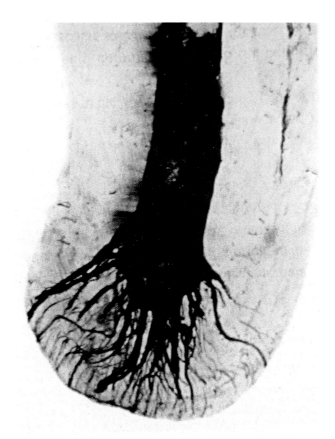

**FIGURE 6-30** Photomicrograph of the apical delta of a dog's tooth. (From Hernandez SZ, Negro VB, Maresca BM. Morphologic features of the root canal system of the maxillary fourth premolar and the mandibular first molar in dogs, *J Vet Dent,* 18:9–13, 2001.)

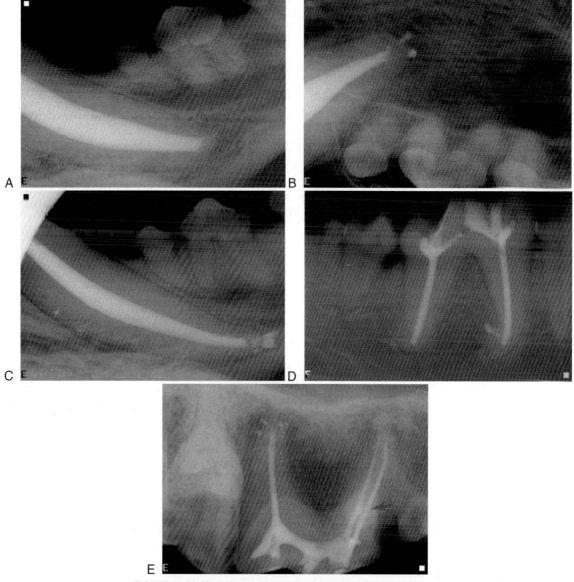

**FIGURE 6-31** The three-dimensional anatomy sometimes only reveals itself after the canals are filled with radiodense obturating materials. **A,** Apical delta on a mandibular canine tooth. **B, C,** Obturating material has filled the apical delta and extruded through canaliculi into the apical periodontal ligament. **D,** A lateral canal is identified due to extruded obturating material. **E,** Apical canals on the distal root and an area of internal resorption on the palatal root (*arrow*).

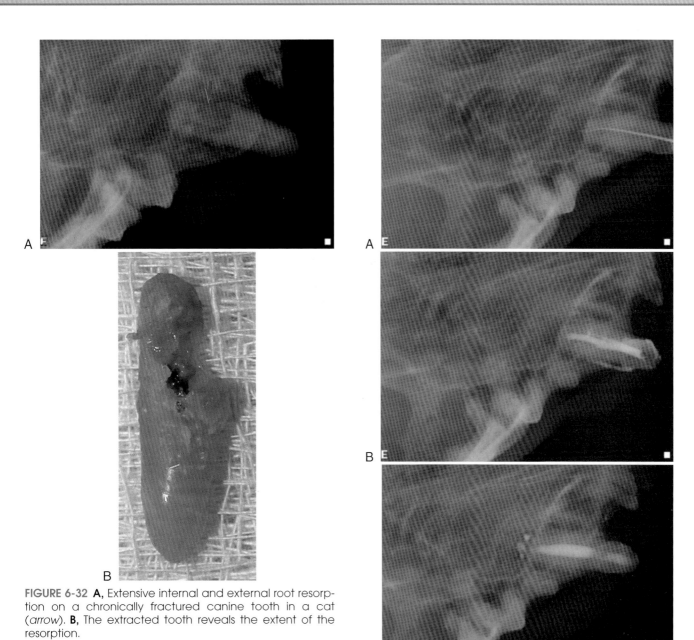

**FIGURE 6-32 A,** Extensive internal and external root resorption on a chronically fractured canine tooth in a cat (*arrow*). **B,** The extracted tooth reveals the extent of the resorption.

**FIGURE 6-33 A,** Open apical foramen in a cat from root tip resorption caused by endodontic inflammation. The file extends through the apex. **B,** Endodontic treatment after creating a positive stop. **C,** The final fill.

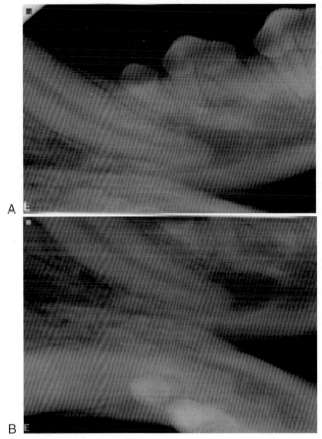

FIGURE 6-34 **A,** Periapical lucency affecting a left mandibular canine tooth that suffered pulp hemorrhage. **B,** The owners did not treat the tooth, and 5 years later there is progression of periapical radiographic pathology that seems less significant than one might expect.

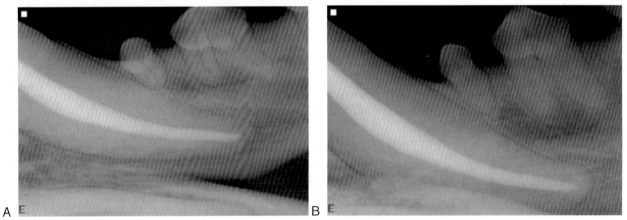

FIGURE 6-35 **A,** Postoperative radiograph of root canal procedure on left mandibular canine tooth. **B,** Two years later the bone has healed and the periodontal ligament is reestablished.

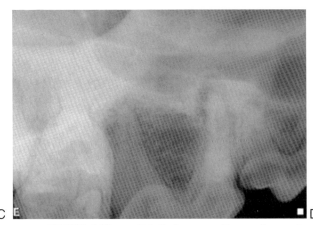
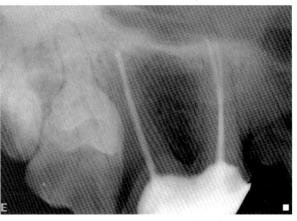

C

D

**FIGURE 6-35, cont'd  C,** Preoperative radiograph of root canal procedure on a right maxillary fourth premolar tooth. **D,** Two years later, the bone has healed and the periodontal ligaments have reestablished.

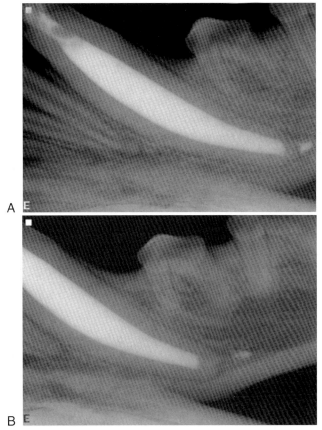

A

B

**FIGURE 6-36** A small amount of extruded sealant should reabsorb over time. However, extruded thermoplasticized gutta percha will not resorb and must be followed radiographically. **A,** The apical blush may be sealant or may include thermosplasticized gutta percha. **B,** Radiograph of the same tooth as in **A** taken 1½ years later. Most of the extruded radiopaque material is gone but some remains.

*Continued.*

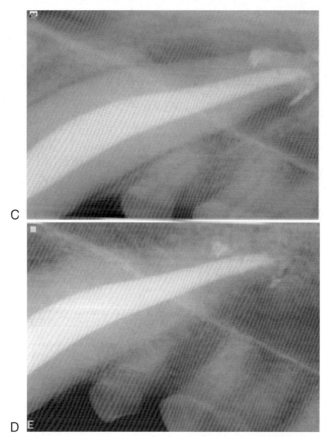

C

D

**FIGURE 6-36, cont'd C,** This is an excessive amount of extruded material. If a surgical approach to debride the periapical tissues and place a root tip filling is not done, it needs to be closely monitored. **D,** This patient was not treated surgically, and follow-up at 3.5 years shows resolution of the bony defect.

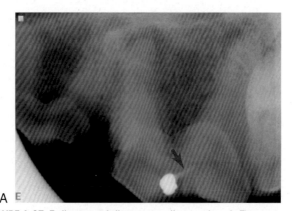

A

**FIGURE 6-37** Failures on follow-up radiographs. **A,** The owner reported that conventional root canal treatment had been performed on the left maxillary fourth premolar tooth. However, none of the roots have been filled and there are periapical radiolucencies. A small piece of gutta percha appears to extend into the distal pulp chamber (*arrow*) under a restoration. The reason for failure is obvious.

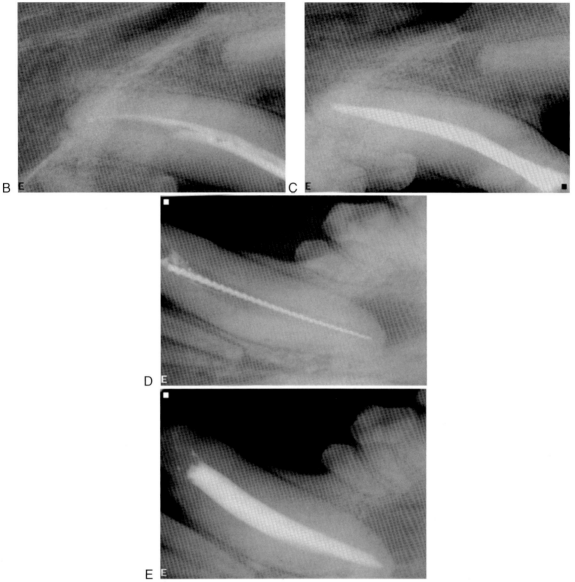

**FIGURE 6-37, cont'd  B,** This right maxillary canine tooth was inadequately obturated. **C,** Retreatment of the tooth in **B** with conventional therapy should resolve the problem. **D,** This mandibular canine tooth had a history of previous root canal treatment years earlier. On the radiograph, there is a broken Hedstrom file, the treatment was not adequately completed, and there is a large periapical lucency. **E,** The file has been removed and the tooth retreated with a conventional endodontic procedure.

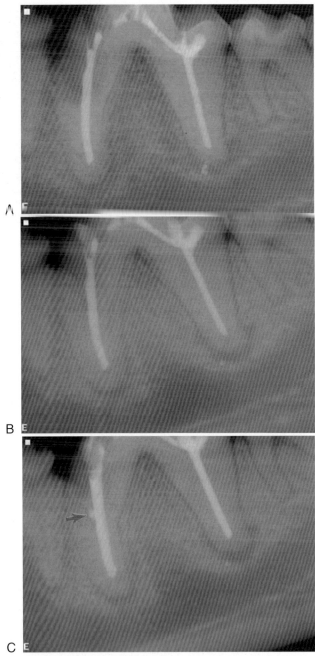

**FIGURE 6-38  A,** Postoperative radiograph of a left mandibular first molar tooth. **B,** Two years later, the periapical lesions have not resolved. In this case, the reason for failure is not obvious. **C,** During retreatment, a tooth resorption can be seen on the mesial root (*arrow*) that was not present or was not filled with sealant during the initial treatment.

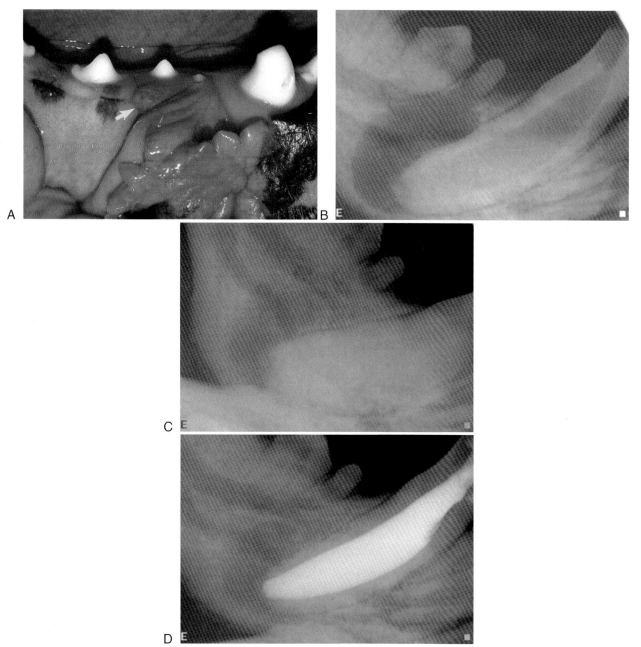

**FIGURE 6-39 A,** A parulis (*arrow*) adjacent to the mandibular second premolar tooth is evidence of an underlying endodontic problem. **B,** The pulp chamber of the canine tooth is large and immature on this 1½-year-old Boxer. This and the large periapical region of bone loss are consistent with pulp necrosis. The apex is open. **C,** Two months after the pulp chamber was cleaned, disinfected, and filled with calcium hydroxide, increased radiopacity indicates mineralization of the periapical lesion. **D,** Now root canal treatment can be performed with a hard tissue stop.

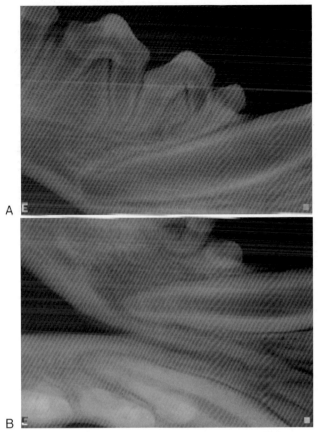

**FIGURE 6-40 A,** Radiograph of an immature canine tooth prior to vital direct pulp cap. **B,** One year later, the apex has closed and the tooth has matured, but then it subsequently failed as evidenced by the periapical lucency. At this point, the tooth needs definitive root canal treatment.

Another endodontic treatment that is sometimes performed in certain circumstances is a vital direct pulp cap. This involves a partial coronal pulpectomy, placement of a medication or material directly on the pulp tissue (usually a mineral trioxide), and a restoration. This has a higher likelihood of failure than routine endodontic treatment and should be monitored with follow-up radiographs 8 to 12 months postoperatively and every 2 to 4 years for the rest of the patient's life to look for evidence of pulp pathosis (Figures 6-40 and 6-41).

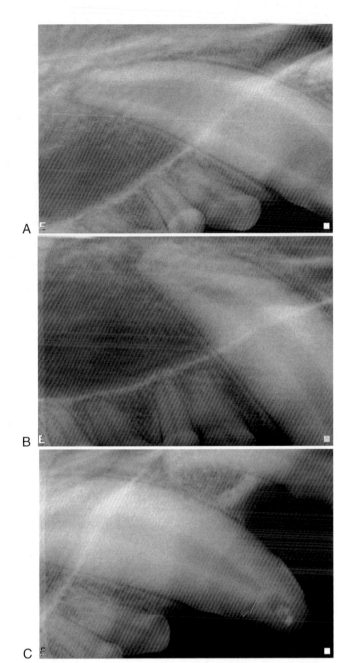

**FIGURE 6-41 A,** Preprocedural radiograph of a maxillary canine tooth treated with vital direct pulp cap. **B,** Eighteen months later, the root canal is narrower, indicating pulp survival and maturation, and the periapical tissues appear healthy but require ongoing monitoring. **C,** On a radiograph of the crown at 18 months posttreatment, a dentin bridge is evident (*arrow*) under the void left behind where calcium hydroxide had been placed. A dentin bridge does not indicate success but merely that the pulp survived long enough to form tertiary, or reparative, dentin.

## SUGGESTED READINGS

Cohen S, Burns RC: *Pathways of the pulp,* ed 6, St. Louis, 1994, Mosby.

Gibilesco JA: *Stafne's oral radiographic diagnosis,* Philadelphia, 1985, WB Saunders.

Jett S, Shrout MK, Mailhot JM, Potter BJ, Borke JL: An evaluation of the origin of trabecular bone patterns using visual and digital image analysis, *Oral Surg Oral Med Oral Pathol Oral Radiol Endod,* 98:598–604, 2004.

Ricucci D, Mannocci F, Pitt Ford TR: A study of periapical lesions correlating the presence of a radiopaque lamina with histological findings, *Oral Surg Oral Med Oral Pathol Oral Radiol Endod,* 101:389–394, 2006.

Stheeman SE, Mileman PA, van der Stelt PF: Diagnostic confidence and the accuracy of treatment decisions for radiopaque periapical lesions, *Int Endod J,* 28:121–128, 1995.

Stock CJR, Gulabivala K, Walker RT, Goodman J: *Color atlas and text of endodontics,* ed 2, London, 1995, Mosby-Wolfe.

Walton RE, Torabinejad M: *Principles and practice of endodontics,* Philadelphia, 1989, WB Saunders.

Whaites E: *Essentials of dental radiography and radiology,* ed 3, New York, 2002, Churchill Livingstone.

# CHAPTER 7

# Tooth Resorption

Resorption of teeth can be a normal physiological process (exfoliation of primary teeth) or a pathological one. Causes of pathological resorption include pressure on the root (impacted tooth or expanding cyst or tumor), inflammation and infection (periodontal, apical, and internal resorption), orthodontic force, trauma (replantation), neoplasia, and after internal bleaching. There is a high incidence of tooth resorption (TR) in cats that are idiopathic, resembling the noncarious cervical tooth resorption seen in dogs, humans, and other species. These are unrelated to cervical lesions that are made by toothbrush abrasion. Although TRs in humans have been called many different terms they are often referred to as "invasive resorption," "idiopathic cervical resorption," and, more recently, "abfraction lesions." The veterinary literature has also given them multiple labels over the years as is common with lesions and syndromes that are poorly understood. Resorption of dental tissue occurs through the action of odontoclasts regardless of the initiating cause, and similar tooth resorption occurs in many different species. Therefore, the term "feline" is inappropriately limiting and the term "odontoclastic" is redundant. For the purposes of this book we will refer to them simply as tooth resorption.

## Feline Tooth Resorption—Clinical Presentations

TRs that have no contact with the oral cavity (do not involve the enamel of the crown or are completely subgingival) are referred to as extraoral and may be present on clinically normal teeth. Extraoral TRs are not associated with discomfort in humans. Supragingival (intraoral) TRs, on the other hand, can cause dental discomfort in people and can be assumed to do the same in cats. Supragingival lesions are readily diagnosed clinically but require radiographs to determine the extent. Mild marginal gingivitis may be the only sign of an early lesion. Sites with localized inflammation should be investigated subgingivally with a sharp dental explorer.

Lesions often appear as though the gingiva is growing up the crown of the tooth due to a tightly adherent gingival or granulomatous tissue (Figure 7-1). This upgrowth of tissue can be quite dramatic, particularly when it occurs on canine teeth (Figure 7-2). Lesions that extend above the gingiva have a sharp enamel margin that is readily identified with an explorer (Figure 7-3). Teeth with small clinical lesions frequently have extensive involvement that can only be identified radiographically (Figure 7-4). TRs can also appear as a missing tooth in an area with a raised alveolar marginal contour or as a pink spot on the crown at the site of internal resorption (Figure 7-5). Gingivitis in the furcation area of a multirooted premolar or molar tooth can mimic a site of resorption. Gingival hyperplasia can mimic the fibrogranulomatous tissue that often fills resorption defects (Figure 7-6). It is important to explore suspicious sites and radiograph the tooth.

Radiographs of affected teeth often show root resorption that is far more advanced than expected. Every tooth with a clinical TR should be radiographically evaluated, not only to determine severity but also to determine the type of root changes that are occurring and to identify concurrent pathology. Multiple teeth are often involved in affected individuals. Therefore, full mouth radiographs of all teeth may be indicated when a patient is diagnosed with TR. Some practitioners recommend full mouth radiographs of all feline patients to identify pathology that is not clinically apparent.

## TYPES

Radiographs of teeth affected with TRs show distinct changes. The roots of some affected teeth seem to "disappear" as they lose radiodense root tissue at a similar rate to the simultaneously occurring osseous repair, effectively making the roots appear to blend with the surrounding bone. The periodontal ligament and structural details are lost. Other TRs retain areas of normal radiodensity interspersed with radiolucencies caused by resorption and do not lose the detail of the periodontal ligament space and root structures in

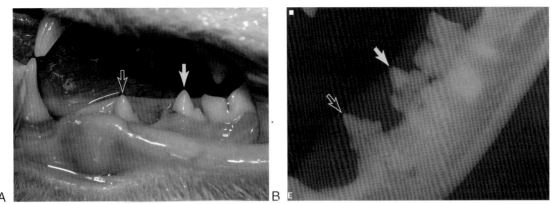

**FIGURE 7-1** **TR on left mandibular fourth premolar tooth (*arrow*). A,** Coronal migration of the mesial gingiva is the only evidence of an underlying problem (bleeding was caused by periodontal probing). There is no intraoral lesion visible and the gingiva is tightly adherent to the tooth. **B,** There is more extensive involvement of the fourth premolar (*arrow*) than clinically suggested with radiolucency of the crown and disruption of the furcation area. The roots of the third premolar tooth (*open arrow*) are also losing radiodensity.

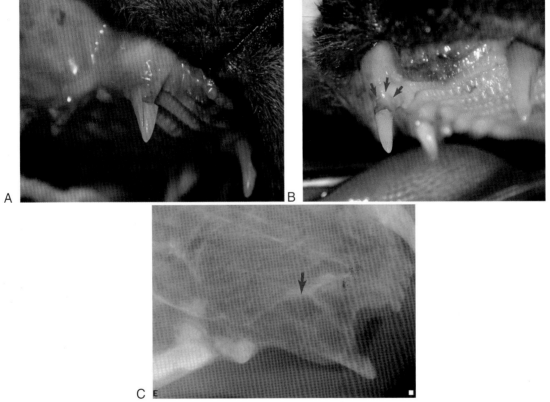

**FIGURE 7-2** **A,** The mesiolabial view of a right maxillary canine tooth in a cat shows extensive damage to the crown and gingival tissue filling a large resorption defect. **B,** On the mesiolingual view of the tooth, the adherent tissue extends far up the crown from the normal position of the gingival margin (*arrows*). **C,** The root and internal crown of the canine tooth is completely resorbed. There is a radiolucency at the site previously occupied by the root (*arrow*). This is consistent with root resorption without evidence of replacement by bone or other hard tissue.

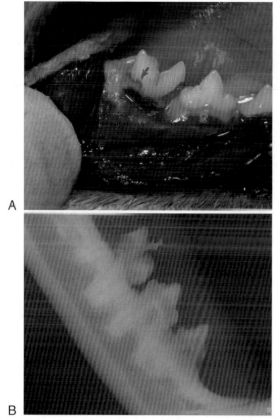

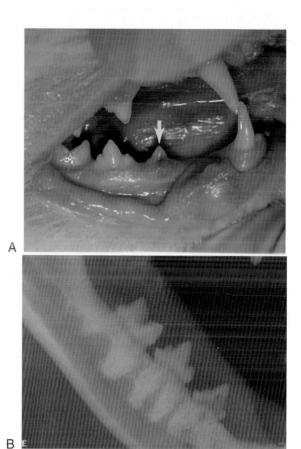

**FIGURE 7-3 A,** TR on the distobuccal surface of a right mandibular molar tooth extends above the gingiva (*arrow*) and does not have adherent tissue in the defect. The margin of the enamel defect can be visualized and can be identified using a dental explorer. The bleeding on the mesial surface was caused by probing. **B,** On a radiograph of the tooth in **A,** a large area of the tooth is destroyed by a tooth resorption (*arrow*).

**FIGURE 7-4 A,** In this patient, TR on the right mandibular third premolar tooth (*arrow*) extends up onto the crown as a deep defect. **B,** On the radiograph, the internal resorption is far more extensive than expected based on the surface lesion.

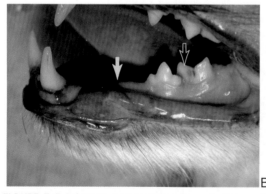

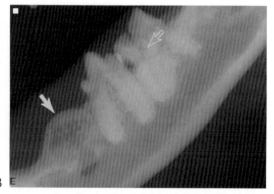

**FIGURE 7-5 Internal crown resorption. A,** This patient is missing the left mandibular third premolar tooth (*arrow*) and has a pink discoloration of the crown of the molar tooth (open arrow). **B,** On the radiograph, there is an end-stage tooth resorption undergoing root replacement at the site of the missing tooth (*arrow*), and the molar tooth has areas of radiolucency in the crown (*open arrow*) and loss of detail of the roots with a regional increase in the alveolar bone opacity.

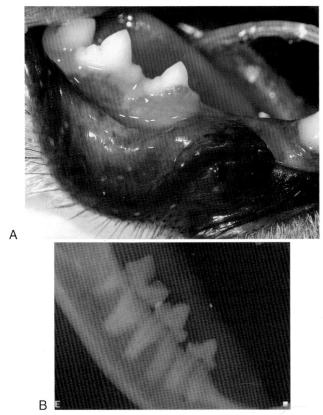

A

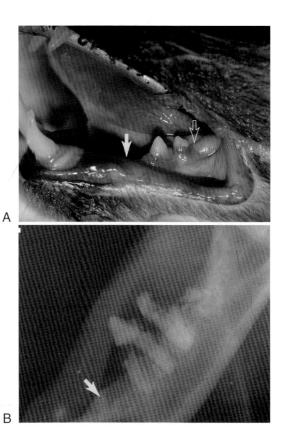

A

B

FIGURE 7-6 **Gingival hyperplasia. A,** The hyperplastic gingiva extending coronally onto the premolar tooth has a similar appearance to the tissue found in tooth resorption. However, in this case, the tissue is not adherent and there is no underlying resorption occurring either clinically or on a radiograph (**B**).

FIGURE 7-7 **Type 1 TRs. A,** The left mandibular third premolar tooth is missing (*arrow*). The gingiva extends coronally on the mesial (rostral) surface of the fourth premolar tooth. The distal (caudal) half of the crown is missing from the molar tooth (*open arrow*). **B,** On the radiograph there are large type 1 TRs on the fourth premolar and molar teeth. Unresorbed areas of the roots are not losing detail or radiopacity. Resorbed areas are not being replaced by bone-dense tissue. A root tip from the missing third premolar tooth is present (*arrow*). It has lost some radiopacity, but the periodontal ligament space is clearly visible and intact.

those areas not directly undergoing resorption. Areas of root resorption are often patchy, remaining radiolucent because the lost root substance is not replaced by reparative tissue. This type of TR also commonly demonstrates concurrent periodontal or endodontic disease.

It is not known if the dissimilarity between the two types is caused by different etiologies, or if it is a result of inflammation interfering with bone repair and tissue replacement, or if some other physiological process acts on one type of lesion but not the other. However, the differences are radiographically detectable and may become important in the search for the etiology and pathophysiology of TRs. Lesions in which the roots are not replaced by bone-dense tissue are termed type 1 lesions (Figures 7-7 through 7-10), while those in which the roots are replaced and appear to disappear are type 2 lesions (Figure 7-11). Both types of lesion can be found in the same individual cat, and even in the same tooth with one root appearing to be type 1 and the other root appearing to be a type 2 (Figure 7-12). It is unknown if this is a stage of severity in which the root or region with the appearance of a type 1 lesion might have eventually progressed to become a type 2 lesion.

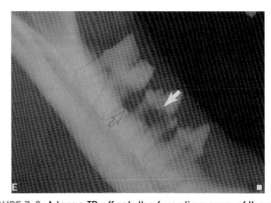

FIGURE 7-8 A large TR affects the furcation area of the right mandibular fourth premolar tooth (*arrow*), and a smaller one is present on the mesial root of the molar tooth. Note the apical position of the alveolar margin (*open arrow*). This alveolar bone loss is a common feature in the bone around teeth with type 1 lesions in contrast to a coronal displacement with type 2 lesions (see Figure 7-5).

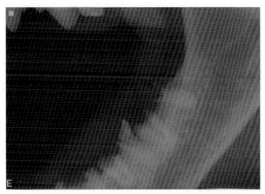

**FIGURE 7-9** Even in very chronic end-stage type 1 lesions, tooth roots remain intact with no evidence of replacement.

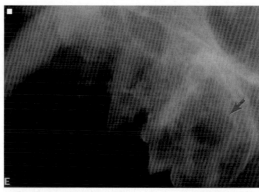

**FIGURE 7-10 Variation of type 1 TR.** The left maxillary premolar teeth are losing radiopacity, but in a patchy and uneven manner. Unaffected areas remain more opaque than the surrounding bone and the periodontal ligament space remains identifiable. The distal root of the fourth premolar tooth is completely gone. There has been no replacement of the lost root material, leaving a distinct radiolucency (*arrow*).

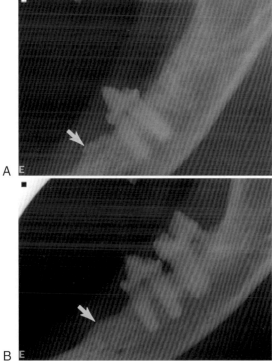

**FIGURE 7-11 Type 2 TRs. A,** The left mandible of this cat is missing the third premolar tooth and the molar tooth. The fourth premolar tooth appears normal. The alveolar bone at the site of the missing premolar is slightly irregular and exhibits a marked positive marginal contour (*arrow*). A faint outline of both resorbed roots of the molar tooth are still identifiable. All root sites have attained a radiopacity similar to that of the surrounding alveolar bone. These characteristics are typical of type 2 lesions. **B,** The left mandibular third premolar tooth is missing (*arrow*). There is no evidence of the previous roots or dental alveoli, and the bony trabeculation appears normal. This is identifiable as an end-stage type 2 lesion only because of the convex elevation of the alveolar marginal bone at the site of the missing tooth. If the tooth were previously extracted or lost to periodontal disease, there would be loss of alveolar vertical dimension with a concave depression rather than an elevation of the bone.

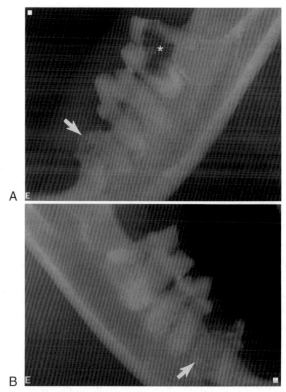

**FIGURE 7-12 Combined type 1 and type 2 TRs. A,** The left mandibular third premolar tooth (*arrow*) has a stage 4 TR that is a type 2 lesion. The radiodensity of the roots is becoming similar to that of the surrounding bone. The molar tooth in the same cat also has a stage 4 TR (*asterisk*), but this one is a type 1 lesion. The roots have normal opacity and an intact periodontal ligament. **B,** The right mandibular third premolar tooth has characteristics of both type 1 and type 2 lesions. The mesial root has maintained normal opacity, while the distal root (*arrow*) is less radiopaque.

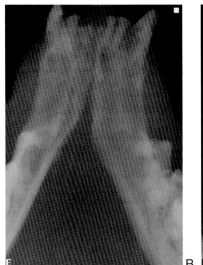 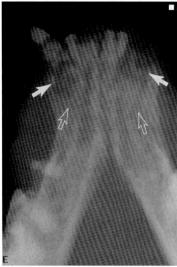

**FIGURE 7-13 A,** This patient presented with stage 4 TRs on both mandibular canine teeth and type 1 TRs on three incisor teeth. The teeth were not extracted. **B,** Two years later, the left canine tooth fractured and the patient was presented for treatment. Radiolucency has developed around the base of the crowns (*arrows*), indicating pathology that must be removed, but the apical sections of resorbed roots remain radiographically quiet (*open arrows*).

Anecdotally, maxillary premolar and molar teeth seem to be more commonly affected by type 1 lesions, whereas mandibular premolar and molar teeth seem to have a higher prevalence of type 2 lesions.

Tooth resorption on the canine teeth of cats often have areas that appear to be combined type 1 and type 2. Over time it becomes more evident on radiographs which areas will be replaced and which are associated with pathology (Figures 7-13 through 7-15).

## STAGES

There are a number of staging systems in the literature for recording the severity or extent of lesions. Of these, the most logical and clear one categorizes TRs by severity according to objective and easily determined observation that places them into stages that may have clinical relevance (see Figures 7-16 and 7-17):

- *Stage 1.* A lesion that affects only the cementum and/or marginal enamel but does not involve the dentin. This stage occurs subgingivally where the tooth surface is exposed to cells that can become odontoclasts. It is uncommon to identify TRs at this stage. Stage 1 lesions are not radiographically apparent.
- *Stage 2.* A lesion that involves the dentin but not the pulp. It can be difficult to know when the pulp is "involved" because shallow dentin lesions bleed readily from their deep margins even when the depth of the lesion is not close to the pulp chamber. This may be due to the rapid spread of resorption through dentin or to internal resorption from the pulp outward to the surface defect (see Figure 7-14).

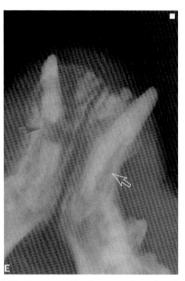

**FIGURE 7-14 Both mandibular canine teeth have root resorption.** The right canine has a mid-root lucency (*arrow*) that does not show evidence of bone replacement. The alveolus is expanded and there is evidence of periodontitis and alveolitis. Both segments of this tooth should be extracted and the tissues debrided and flushed prior to surgical closure. The left canine tooth has a vertical root lucency (*open arrow*) that has the appearance of an early type 2 TR.

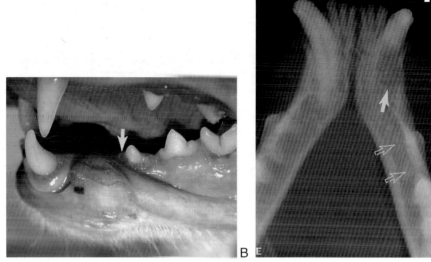

**FIGURE 7-15 Feline TRs on canine teeth. A,** This cat has a swollen lip in the area of the frenulum. There is a TR (*arrow*) on the left mandibular third premolar tooth. The canine tooth appears normal. **B,** The lesion on the premolar is a quiet type 2 TR (*open arrow*) that requires a standard premolar projection to properly evaluate (see Chapter 12). The canine tooth has a large periapical lucency and loss of the root with no replacement (*arrow*). On surgical examination, the defect was filled with purulent material.

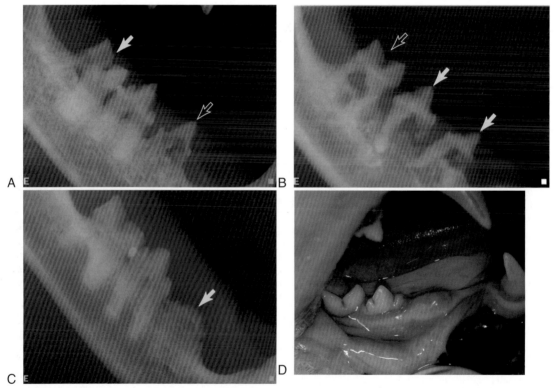

**FIGURE 7-16 Stages of TRs. A,** The right mandibular molar tooth (*arrow*) has a stage 3 (type 1) lesion. The third premolar tooth (*open arrow*) has a stage 4 (type 2) lesion. **B,** The third and fourth premolar teeth (*arrows*) have stage 4 lesions. The molar tooth (*open arrow*) has a stage 3 lesion. All are type 1. **C,** The type 2 lesion on this right mandibular third premolar tooth (*arrow*) may be a stage 4 or 5 depending on whether there is any tooth not completely covered by gingiva. This cannot be determined radiographically. **D,** A photograph of the quadrant radiographed in **C** shows that the gingiva covers the entire hard tissue, making this a stage 5 lesion.

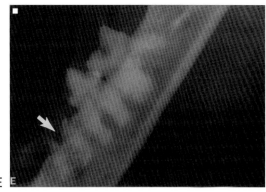

FIGURE 7-16, cont'd **E,** Stage 5 (type 1) lesion (*arrow*).

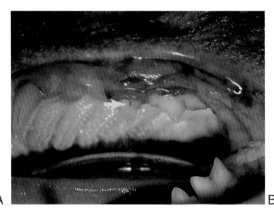
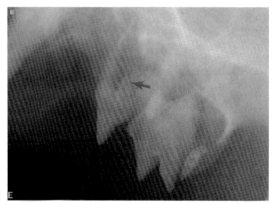

FIGURE 7-17 **A,** This lesion (*arrow*) appears to be a stage 2 lesion on clinical examination—clearly through the enamel but extending only slightly into the dentin. **B,** The radiograph of the tooth in **A** shows a vertical lucency (*arrow*) of the distal root, indicating resorption and deeper involvement than was clinically apparent.

- *Stage 3.* A lesion that involves the pulp. Lesions often spare the pulp and peripulpal dentin. Radiographs may be necessary to evaluate pulp involvement.
- *Stage 4.* A lesion that has destroyed a significant amount of the crown, weakening the crown and placing it at risk of fracture with only moderate trauma.
- *Stage 5.* A lesion that has destroyed the entire crown of the tooth. The gingiva has grown over the roots and no tooth material is exposed to the oral cavity.

Radiographic evaluation allows both the type and stage of a lesion to be determined, both of which can be easily recorded on the patient's dental chart.

## Tooth Resorption in Dogs

Similar to cats and other species, dogs are affected by TRs from both known causes (most commonly periodontal or endodontic infection or inflammation) (Figure 7-18) and from unproved etiology. The (currently) idiopathic TRs are far less prevalent than the feline lesions and appear very similar to the idiopathic type of TRs in cats (Figure 7-19). Type 1, type 2, and combined TRs are found in dogs, and they can be staged using the same criteria that are used to stage feline TRs. As in feline lesions, radiographs often show much more severe tooth involvement than is seen clinically, sometimes affecting teeth that have no apparent intraoral defects (Figure 7-20). TRs in dogs also act clinically similar to TRs in cats making restoration a poor treatment choice. Even after endodontic treatment and restoration, a lesion can continue to progress if the restoration extends subgingivally or close enough to the gingival margin to allow the gingiva to reach it and to provide a source of odontoclasts.

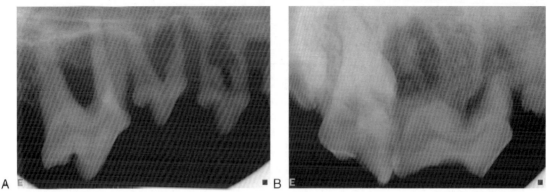

**FIGURE 7-18** **Dental tooth resorption in dogs—known etiology. A,** Root resorption caused by periodontal infection (see Chapter 5) The roots of the right maxillary second and third premolar teeth have multiple tooth resorptions in areas of alveolar bone loss. (From DuPont GD, DeBowes LJ: Comparison of periodontitis and root replacement in cat teeth with resorptive lesions, *J Vet Dent,* 19: 71–75, 2002.) **B,** Root resorption caused by endodontic disease. The right maxillary fourth premolar tooth has extensive root resorption caused by inflammatory mediators that have escaped from the endodontic system with a necrotic pulp (see Chapter 6).

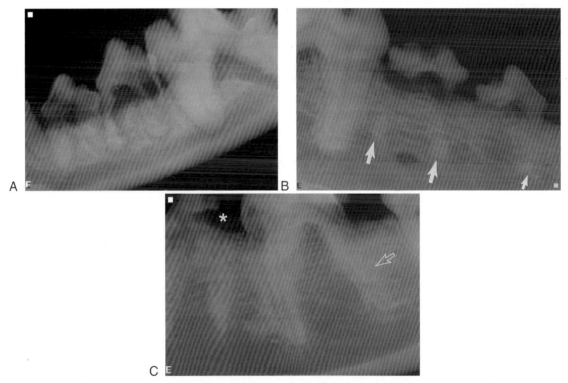

**FIGURE 7-19** **Types of ideopathic TR in dog teeth. A,** Multiple type 1 lesions on the mandibular third and fourth premolar teeth of a dog. **B,** Multiple type 2 lesions on the mandibular third and fourth premolar teeth of a dog. Three of the root tips are not resorbing at the same rate (*arrows*) and need to be monitored. **C,** Combined lesions. Most of the left mandibular fourth premolar tooth crown is missing (*asterisk*). The mesial root (*left*) appears completely replaced, and the distal root nearly so. The first molar tooth appears most like a type 1 lesion with normal radiodensity and patchy radiolucencies. However, some areas of the distal root appear to be undergoing replacement like a type 2 lesion (*open arrow*).

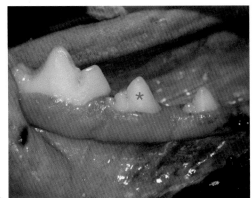

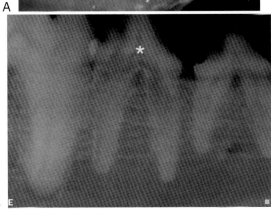

FIGURE 7-20 **A,** Clinically normal right mandibular fourth premolar tooth (*asterisk*). **B,** Just as in cats, the radiographic appearance often reveals more extensive involvement than clinically evident from examining the tooth crown.

## SUGGESTED READINGS

Benenati FW: Root resorption: Types and treatment, *Gen Dent,* 45:42–45, 1997.

Frank AL: Extracanal invasive resorption: An update, *Comp Cont Educ Dent,* 16:250–254, 1995.

Gengler W, Dubielzig R, Ramer J: Physical examination and radiographic analysis to detect dental and mandibular bone resorption in cats: A study of 81 cases from necropsy, *J Vet Dent,* 12:97–100, 1995.

Gorrel C, Larsson A: Feline odontoclastic resorptive lesions: unveiling the early lesion, *J Small Anim Pract,* 43:482–488, 2002.

Heimisdottir K, Bosshardt D, Ruf S: Can the severity of root resorption be accurately judged by means of radiographs? A case report with histology, *Am J Orthod Dentofac Orthop,* 128:106–109, 2005.

Heithersay GS: Clinical, radiologic, and histopathologic features of invasive cervical resorption, *Quintessence Int,* 30:27-37, 1999.

Kuroe T, Itoh H, Caputo AA, et al: Biomechanics of cervical tooth structure lesions and their restoration, *Quintessence Int,* 31:267–274, 2000.

Okuda A, Harvey CE: Etiopathogenesis of feline dental resorptive lesions. In Harvey CE (ed): *Feline Dentistry, Vet Clin North Am Small Anim Pract,* 22:1385, 1992.

Trope M: Root resorption of dental origin: Classification based on etiology, *Pract Periodont Aesthet Dent,* 10:515–522, 1998.

Verstraete FJ, Kass PH, Terpak CH: Diagnostic value of full-mouth radiography in cats, *Am J Vet Res,* 59:692–695, 1998.

# CHAPTER 8

# Swelling and Neoplasia

Some common causes of oral swelling include
- Endodontic infection (see Chapter 6)
- Developmental abnormality (see Chapter 9)
- Trauma (see Chapter 10)
- Periodontal abscess and pyogenic granuloma (see Chapter 5)
- Infection
- Cyst
- Benign tumor
- Neoplasia

## Infection and Inflammation

Infections can result in oral swelling caused by inflammation or fluid accumulation. Infected root or bone fragments that persist after a tooth is lost are a common cause of swelling. Penetrating wounds or foreign bodies can also introduce bacteria into the deep oral tissues. Periodontal infections usually have adequate sulcular drainage to prevent swelling, but a periodontal abscess can occur if this outlet is blocked. Even with adequate drainage, a localized gingival swelling can occur in the form of a pyogenic granuloma. Focal fibrous hyperplasia can become large enough to mimic gingival tumors (Figure 8-1). Many of the lesions classified as fibromatous epulides are very likely fibrous hyperplasia. Endodontic infections can also present as swollen tissues if they are unable to establish drainage along the root or through a fistulous tract. A small localized swelling (parulis) can develop where a draining tract exits or is about to break open. When infection spreads from the initial site through the marrow spaces, it establishes osteomyelitis. This can manifest as an oral swelling (Figure 8-2) but can also occur with minimal or no tissue enlargement (see Chapter 11).

## Oral and Dental Cysts

There are a multitude of cysts that occur in the oral cavity, of which only a few odontogenic cysts with radiographic significance are included.

Apical radicular cysts (also called apical periodontal cysts, periapical cysts, and radicular cysts) are related to pulp inflammation or necrosis and are discussed in Chapter 6.

Lateral radicular cysts (sometimes called lateral periodontal cysts) are a type of odontogenic cyst that originates either from remnants of the Hertzwig epithelial root sheath (epithelial rests of Malassez) along the side of a root or possibly from remnants of dental lamina, which would make them similar in origin to adult gingival cysts (Figure 8-3). They are asymptomatic and often discovered late after they have attained a significant size, expanding the bone both labially and toward the nasal cavity (Figure 8-4). The most commonly identified lateral radicular cysts are associated with the maxillary canine teeth of dogs. Most are unilocular radiolucent lesions, but rarely there is a polycystic variant. Surgical debridement of the cyst lining with retention of the affected tooth is curative.

The dentigerous cyst is one type of odontogenic cyst called a follicular cyst that is an epithelium-lined sac surrounding the crown of an unerupted tooth. The epithelium is attached at the cervical area of the tooth. An eruption cyst (eruption hematoma) is a dentigerous cyst that is close to the surface surrounding a tooth that is eventually able to erupt, either naturally or with a minor operculectomy surgery or removal of the roof of the cyst (Figure 8-5). The tissue covering the teeth sometimes includes bone, in which case the redundant gingiva as well as the bone should be surgically removed to facilitate further tooth eruption. Deeper dentigerous cysts that surround an impacted tooth or one in which eruption has been irreversibly interrupted are relatively common, particularly associated with mandibular first premolar teeth (Figure 8-6). It can also occur with maxillary first premolar teeth and occasionally other teeth as well. Unerupted supernumerary first premolars can cause a cyst under the surface in an area where there is no tooth missing from the erupted dentition (Figure 8-7). Radiographs are not diagnostic for dentigerous cysts because odontogenic keratocysts, unilocular ameloblastomas, and other lesions may appear similar on radiographs. Dentigerous cysts often

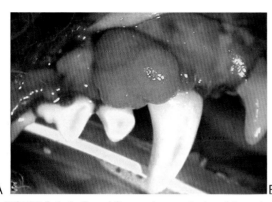
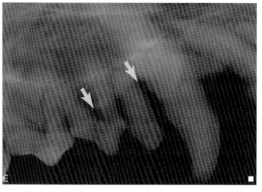

A          B

FIGURE 8-1 **A,** Focal fibrous hyperplasia of the gingiva adjacent to the canine and premolar teeth. **B,** Radiograph of the patient in **A.** Loss of alveolar marginal bone (*arrows*) caused by periodontitis. The local inflammation stimulated the benign tissue hyperplasia.

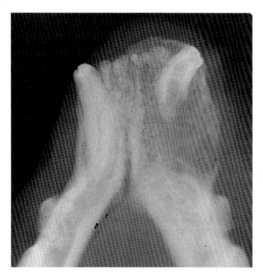

FIGURE 8-2 **Osteomyelitis in a cat mandible.** The left mandibular canine tooth has a fractured crown with chronic pulp necrosis. The pulp chamber is wide and there is external resorption of the root tip. The bone is characterized by generalized enlargement and radiolucency. Osteomyelitis can appear radiographically similar to neoplasia, particularly in cats.

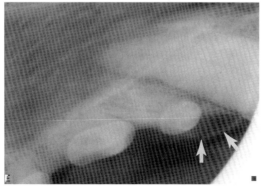

FIGURE 8-3 **Lateral radicular cyst.** On an occlusal projection, the labial bone is elevated from the root of the canine tooth (*arrows*).

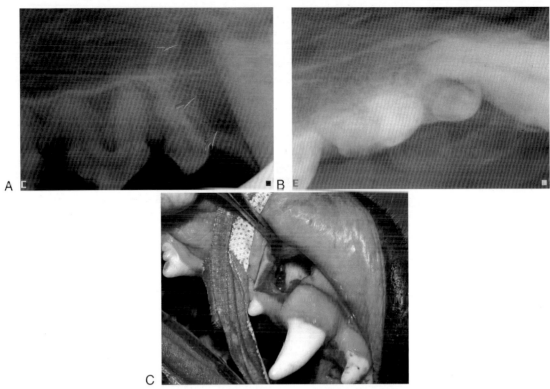

**FIGURE 8-4 Lateral radicular cyst.** In this patient, the cyst extended along the labial, distal, and palatal surfaces of the canine tooth root. **A,** On a standard radiograph, the defect involved most of the distal surface (*arrows*). **B,** On an occlusal view, the labial extension adjacent to the first premolar tooth can be appreciated. **C,** Surgical exposure of the defect reveals a denuded root surface.

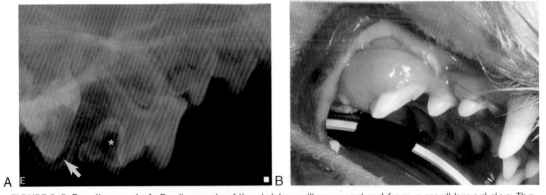

**FIGURE 8-5 Eruption cyst. A,** Radiograph of the right maxillary quadrant from a small-breed dog. The cap of the fourth maxillary deciduous premolar tooth is present (*asterisk*). There is a radiolucent line surrounding the crown of the unerupted first molar tooth surrounded by a radiopaque line (*arrow*). This is an eruption cyst of an embedded molar that is encased in maxillary bone. **B,** The fourth premolar tooth has erupted but the gingival contour has not receded to its normal position. Gingivectomy to remove the pseudopocket and restore a normal gingival architecture accelerates a return to normal. This patient is also missing the first premolar tooth.

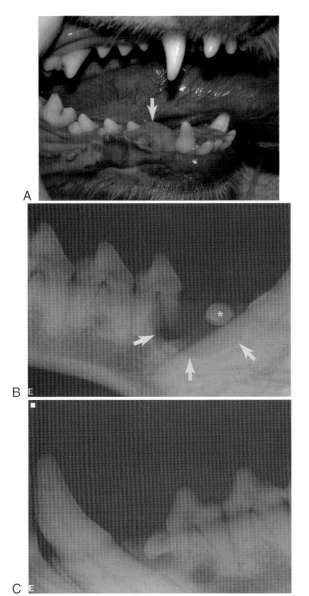

A

B

C

**FIGURE 8-6 Dentigerous cyst. A,** There is a fluctuant dark blue swelling in the area of the missing right mandibular first premolar tooth (*arrow*). **B,** On a radiograph of the dog in **A,** there is an axial view of the unerupted buccolingually oriented first premolar tooth (*asterisk*). A circular lucency surrounds the tooth (*arrows*) indicating a dentigerous cyst. The mesial root of the second premolar is shortened due to interruption of development, pressure resorption, or both. **C,** The contralateral (*left*) mandibular first premolar tooth on the same patient is also developing a dentigerous cyst.

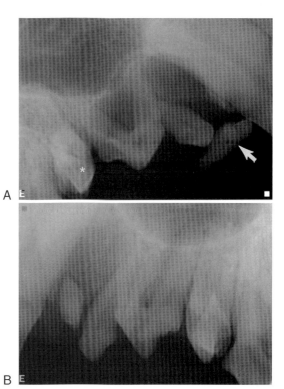

A

B

**FIGURE 8-7 Dentigerous cyst of a supernumerary tooth. A,** One of the first premolar teeth sits sideways and appears to float in the lucency of the cyst it has caused (*arrow*). The third premolar tooth is rotated 90 degrees (*asterisk*), a common finding in brachycephalic dogs. **B,** The radiograph of the left quadrant of the same patient reveals an unerupted supernumerary first premolar on this side also. There is no radiographic evidence of overt cyst formation, but the entire periodontal ligament appears abnormally wide.

found in any breed. Many unerupted first premolar teeth remain quiet throughout life and do not develop dentigerous cysts (Figure 8-9).

Dentigerous cysts of multiple teeth can occur when there is an interruption in the general eruption process (Figure 8-10).

The origin of an odontogenic cyst is not always immediately apparent, and in these cases the patient should be monitored for recurrence.

Odontogenic cysts also occur in cats (Figure 8-11).

## Oral Tumors

The many different types of tumors found in the oral cavity arise from the soft tissues, from the bone, or from the teeth themselves. Not all neoplastic processes manifest as swelling or mass lesions. They may present as a single tooth or group of teeth exhibiting mobility in an otherwise healthy mouth or as delayed healing after extraction or surgery. Therefore, it is prudent to obtain radiographs of the regional supportive bone and send tissue samples for histopathology evaluation in these cases even in the absence of swelling. Included here

remain undiagnosed for many years, allowing them to become quite large, dissecting along the mandible, where they can interfere with the development and cause pressure resorption of the roots of other teeth in the quadrant (Figure 8-8). In early lesions, the crown often projects into the defect. Later, as the cyst changes location, the crown may no longer be within the lucency. Brachycephalic dog breeds seem to be predisposed to this, although they can be

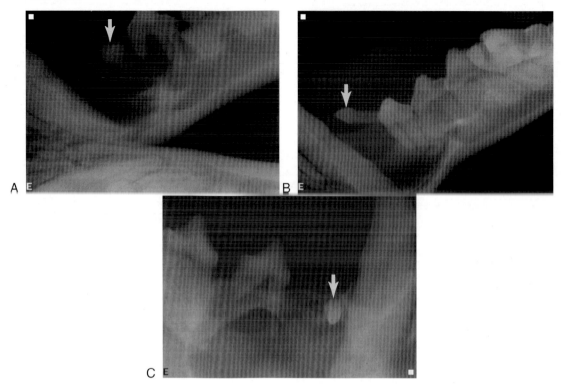

**FIGURE 8-8 Extensive dentigerous cysts.** Each of these was caused by an unerupted first premolar tooth (*arrows*). **A,** Pressure from the expanding cyst has damaged bone to the level of the distal root of the second premolar tooth. **B,** The bone loss extends to the third premolar tooth. **C,** A very large and expansile cyst has a multiloculated appearance.

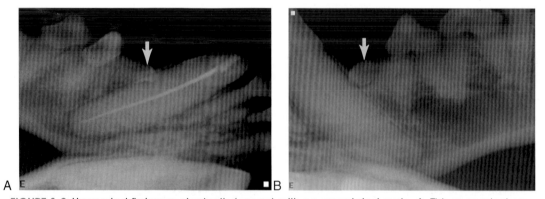

**FIGURE 8-9 Unerupted first premolar teeth (*arrows*) with no associated cysts. A,** This unerupted premolar tooth was found as an incidental finding on radiographs made during endodontic treatment. **B,** An unerupted tooth on a 12-year-old Lhasa Apso.

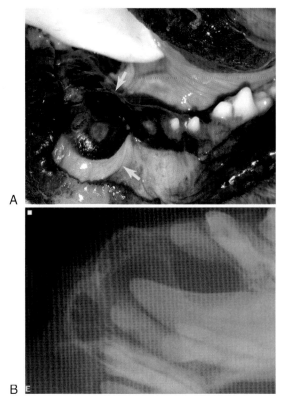

**FIGURE 8-10 Multiple unerupted teeth.** This dog's left mandibular incisor, canine, and rostral premolar teeth never erupted. She also had a marked mandibular distoclusion ("underbite"). The gingival swelling around the site of the missing canine tooth (*arrows*) had recently begun to enlarge. **B,** The radiograph of the patient in **A** is characterized by multiple unerupted teeth with dentigerous cyst formation.

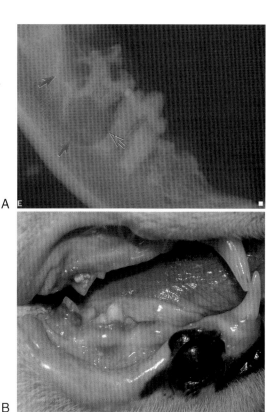

**FIGURE 8-11 Odontogenic cysts in a cat. A,** Tooth resorptions are present on the right mandibular molar tooth. The periapical regions of both roots of the molar have large radiolucencies (*arrows*) and there is evidence of pressure resorption on the distal root of the fourth premolar tooth (*open arrowhead*). The third premolar tooth is missing (stage 5 type 2 tooth resorption; see Chapter 7) and the alveolar margin at the resorption site has an irregular border. **B,** Fluctuant blue swellings adjacent to the molar, fourth premolar, and missing third premolar are evidence of shallow underlying cysts. The cyst lumens contained keratin and the surrounding bone exhibited compression osteolysis on histopathology. The osteolysis is radiographically visible in the molar area but not the premolar area.

are a few of the oral tumors with emphasis on those that cause radiographic changes.

## BENIGN TUMORS

### Fibroma

Fibromas are soft tissue lesions that generally have no associated radiographic abnormalities. Some of the lesions that are reported as "fibromatous epulides" are very likely fibromas.

The peripheral odontogenic fibroma is a lesion that, along with the fibroma and fibrous hyperplasia, is often classified as a "fibromatous epulis." These tumors also have no radiographic signs in early lesions. As the lesion progresses, affected bone enlarges and teeth are displaced (Figure 8-12, *A*). Peripheral odontogenic fibromas are also sometimes classified as "fibromatous and ossifying epulis" and as "ossifying epulis," depending on the degree of mineralization (Figure 8-12, *B*). Focal inflammatory lesions can sometimes mimic peripheral odontogenic fibromas in dogs (see Figure 8-1) and in cats (Figure 8-13).

The peripheral ossifying fibroma may also be classified as an ossifying epulis. It looks clinically the same as a peripheral odontogenic fibroma, both affecting the marginal gingiva. Peripheral ossifying fibromas may be reactive lesions rather than neoplastic lesions. They arise from fibrous connective tissue of the periodontal ligament and later mineralize.

Amyloblastoma is an odontogenic tumor. The canine acanthomatous ameloblastoma is a locally invasive tumor that, unlike the peripheral ameloblastoma in humans, aggressively invades the bone. This tumor is often called "acanthomatous epulis" (Figure 8-14).

Amyloblastoma is much less common in cats. They appear radiographically as a radiolucency in the alveolar bone that is associated with a root or possibly an unerupted crown (Figure 8-15).

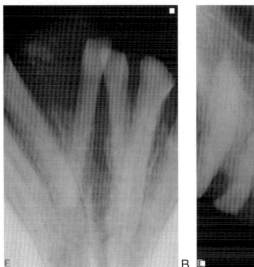
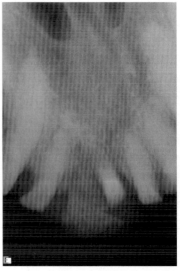

**FIGURE 8-12 Peripheral odontogenic fibroma. A,** The right mandibular first and second incisor teeth crowns are pushed away from each other by a mass between them that has the radiodensity of soft tissue with focal mineralization. **B,** This tumor is pushing apart the right maxillary first and second incisor teeth. Mineralized tissues in the tumor are visible as radiodense tissue.

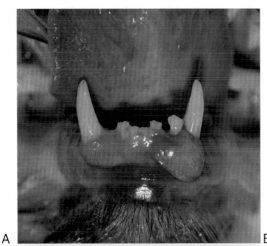
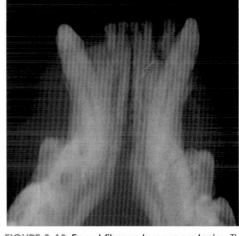
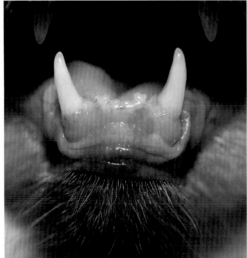

**FIGURE 8-13 Focal fibrous hyperperplasia.** The histopathological diagnosis was feline fibromatous epulis. **A,** The firm enlargement of tissue around the left mandibular third incisor tooth extended labial to the canine tooth. **B,** There is loss of bony support for the incisor tooth (*arrow*). **C,** The tissues of the patient in **A** appear normal one month after incisional biopsy, extraction of the incisor tooth and curettage.

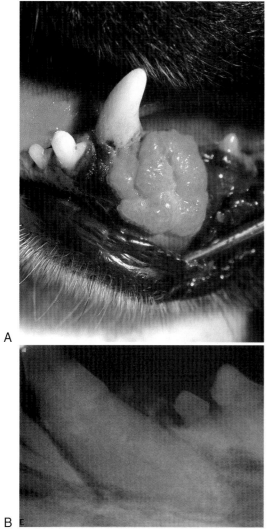

**FIGURE 8-14 Canine acanthomatous ameloblastoma.**
**A,** Firm proliferative mass involves the tissues labial to the left mandibular canine tooth. **B,** Bony destruction results in an area of relative radiolucency in the affected area (*arrows*).

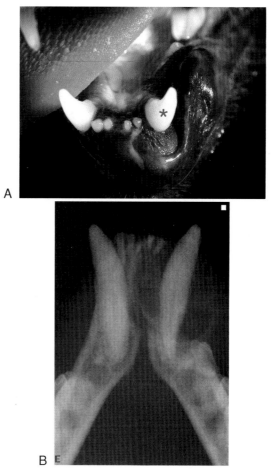

**FIGURE 8-15** **Amyloblastoma in a cat. A,** This cat has an amyloblastoma associated with the left mandibular canine tooth (*asterisk*). The swelling is deviating the lip labially. **B,** The lucency in the radiograph has the "soap bubble" appearance typical of a conventional amyloblastoma; the most common type in humans.

The calcifying epithelial odontogenic tumor (also referred to as an amyloid-producing odontogenic tumor or Pindborg's tumor) is similar to the ameloblastoma and presents as a jaw expansion or as an incidental finding on radiographs. It invades through direct extension and does not metastasize (Figure 8-16).

Odontomas are benign hamartomatous lesions consisting of mature enamel and dentin. The enamel and dentin of compound odontomas are arranged similar to normal teeth (dentin on the inside and enamel on the outside) except that the teeth are supernumerary, multiple, deformed, and small (Figure 8-17). They mature at about the same time as the permanent teeth in the area and are not fused with the normal teeth. Anecdotally, they seem overrepresented in some spaniel breeds but are also found in other breeds. Complex

odontomas are arranged with the dental tissues mixed together in a disorganized mixed conglomerate of enamel, dentin, and cementum (Figure 8-18).

## MALIGNANT TUMORS

Malignant melanoma is considered to be the most common malignant oral neoplasm in the dog but a rare tumor in the cat. It grows rapidly, is very locally invasive, and metastasizes early (Figure 8-19). Involvement of the bone occurs early. The long-term survival rate is not good, particularly for large tumors, because even with adequate margins the rate of metastasis is high.

Squamous cell carcinoma is the second most common malignant neoplasm in dogs and the most common one in cats. It is very locally invasive (Figures 8-20 and 8-21) but

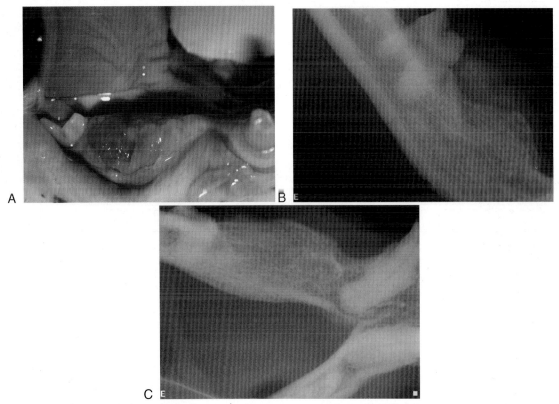

FIGURE 8-16 **Calcifying epithelial odontogenic tumor. A,** Ulceroproliferative tissue covers a firm, enlarged right mandible on a cat. **B,** The entire vertical dimension of the mandible is diffusely involved with a slightly mottled appearance. **C,** In a radiograph made at a more occlusal projection angle, there is evidence of full width involvement extending to the buccal and the lingual surfaces.

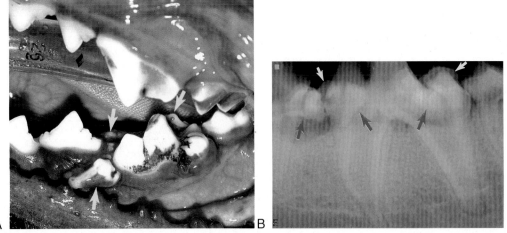

FIGURE 8-17 **Compound odontoma. A,** Rudimentary teeth are positioned mesial, buccal, and lingual to the left mandibular first molar tooth of a dog (*arrows*). **B,** On a radiograph of the patient in **A,** radiodensities (*arrows*) caused by the rudimentary teeth are visible in the interproximal space mesial to the first molar tooth and superimposed over it.

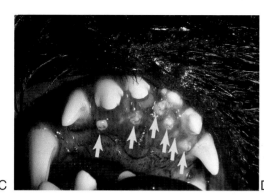
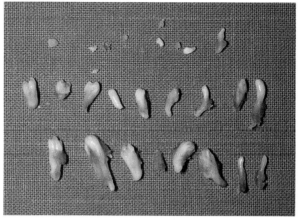

FIGURE 8-17, cont'd  **C,** Multiple rudimentary teeth of a compound odontoma (*arrows*) in the incisor tooth area of a dog. **D,** Multiple small toothlike structures that were removed from a dog with a compound odontoma.

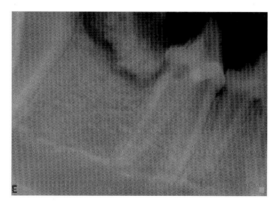

FIGURE 8-18  **Complex odontoma.** A radiopaque mass between the premolar and molar tooth is composed of disorganized dental tissues. The premolar tooth is rotated.

metastasizes slowly. Papillary squamous cell carcinoma in young dogs is distinct from other squamous cell carcinomas in that it has a good prognosis with surgical removal and seems to do well even with conservative surgical margins (Figure 8-22).

Fibrosarcoma is the third most common malignant tumor in dogs and the second most common in cats. It is very locally invasive but has a relatively lower rate of metastasis. The radiographic appearance is variable, ranging from destruction of underlying bone (Figure 8-23) to an increase in bone density. Surgical excision with wide margins is the treatment of choice. Fibrosarcoma is considered to be resistant to radiation therapy, but radiation is possibly an effective adjunctive therapy after surgical removal.

A type of fibrosarcoma known as a histologically low-grade yet biologically high-grade fibrosarcoma occurs in large-breed dogs, often in Golden Retrievers (Figure 8-24). This tumor should be suspected when a histopathology report diagnoses a benign fibromatous appearance on a tumor that is acting clinically aggressive, and it should be treated as a malignancy. They are locally invasive and can metastasize.

Osteosarcoma, the fourth most common malignant tumor of dogs, can cause swelling, pain, and tooth mobility. There is no typical radiographic appearance of osteosarcoma. Early changes include subtle changes in trabeculation. Symmetric widening of periodontal ligaments of multiple teeth in a region can occur from tumor infiltration into the periodontal ligaments. Osteosarcomas can be characterized by destructive lesions with indistinct borders, sclerosis, lysis, or a combination of all. Penetration of the bony lesion into soft tissues can result in the radiographic appearance of trabecular bone radiating out in a "sunburst" effect. Teeth in the area are often characterized by irregular root resorption (Figure 8-25).

Osseous plasma cell tumor is an uncommon tumor (Figure 8-26).

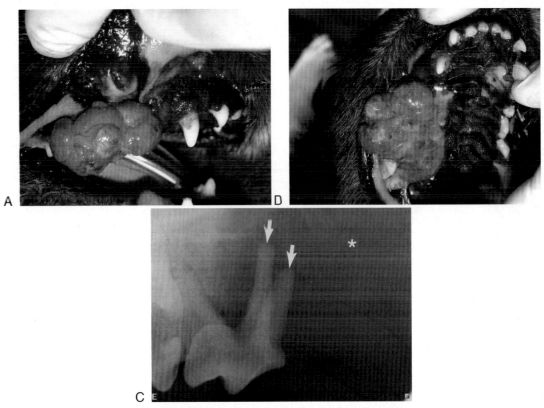

**FIGURE 8-19** **Amelanotic malignant melanoma. A,** Buccal view. **B,** Palatal view reveals the extent of invasion onto the palate. **C,** Extensive loss of bony density in the area of the tumor (*asterisk*). The third premolar tooth is missing and the mesiobuccal and palatal roots of the fourth premolar (*arrows*) appear to "float" in soft tissue.

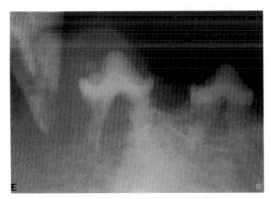

**FIGURE 8-20** **Squamous cell carcinoma in a dog.** Invasion and destruction of the bone is evident as well as resorption of the regional tooth roots.

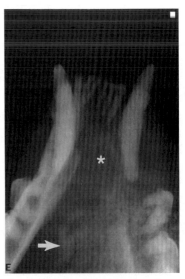

**FIGURE 8-21** **Squamous cell carcinoma in a cat.** The left mandible is characterized by both destructive (*asterisk*) and proliferative (*arrow*) changes.

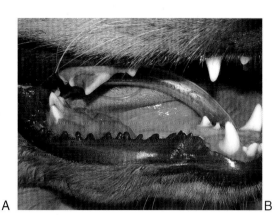
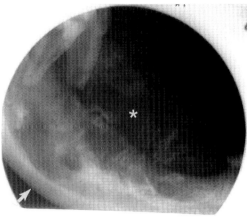

**FIGURE 8-22** **Papillary squamous cell carcinoma in a young dog. A,** This large tumor on the right mandible of a 1-year-old dog first appeared at three months of age. The third and fourth premolars are missing and the first molar is rotated. The initial histopathological diagnosis was "epulis," then squamous cell carcinoma. **B,** There is bony destruction (*asterisk*) and expansion (*arrow*) of the mandible.

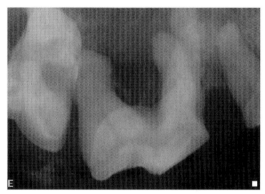

**FIGURE 8-23** **Fibrosarcoma.** In this patient, the tumor is characterized by generalized loss of opacity of the alveolar bone in the affected area.

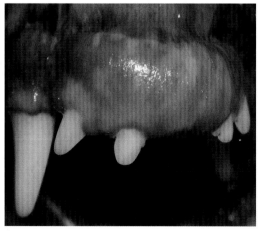
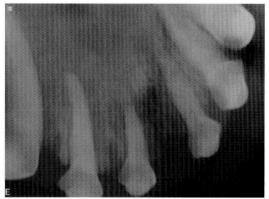

**FIGURE 8-24** **Fibrosarcoma, histologically low-grade and biologically high-grade malignancy. A,** The area of both incisive bones is generally enlarged. The right first incisor tooth was removed with the biopsy sample. **B,** The affected bone is characterized by wide dental septae, attenuation of the apical sections of the roots, and loss of bony trabeculation.

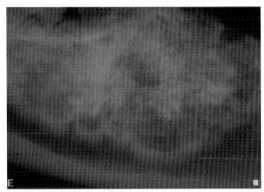

FIGURE 8-25 Osteosarcoma can be characterized by a moth eaten appearance of the bone and irregular root resorption.

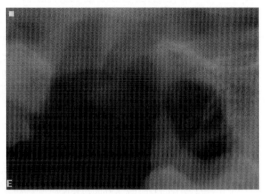

FIGURE 8-26 **Malignant plasma cell tumor.** The radiographic lesion is characterized by a multilocular lytic area with well defined margins.

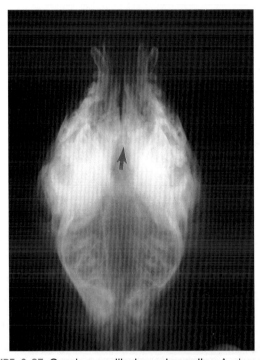

FIGURE 8-27 **Craniomandibular osteopathy.** A dorsoventral view of the skull of a dog with craniomandibular osteopathy is characterized by severe mandibular swelling and obliteration of the intermandibular space (*arrow*).

## Craniomandibular Osteopathy

A less common cause of mandibular swelling is craniomandibular osteopathy, a benign syndrome seen mainly in young terrier breeds. The syndrome is self-limiting, but the changes do not regress. It can cause significant discomfort, salivation, and difficulty prehending food. Mandibular swelling can be extreme, obliterating the rostral intermandibular space (Figure 8-27).

## SUGGESTED READINGS

Gibilesco JA: *Stafne's oral radiographic diagnosis,* Philadelphia, 1985, WB Saunders.

Neville BW, Damm DD, White DK, Waldron CA: *Color atlas of clinical oral pathology,* Philadelphia, 1991, Lea and Febiger.

Regezi JA, Sciubba J: *Oral pathology, clinical-pathologic correlations,* ed 2, Philadelphia, 1993, WB Saunders.

Seguin B: Tumors of the mandible, maxilla, and calvarium. In Slatter D (ed): *Textbook of small animal surgery,* ed 3, Philadelphia, 1993, WB Saunders.

Verstraete JM: Oral pathology. In Slatter D (ed): *Textbook of small animal surgery,* ed 3, Philadelphia, 2002, WB Saunders.

Wiggs RB, Lobprise HB: *Veterinary dentistry principles and practice,* Philadelphia, 1997, Lippincott-Raven.

# Developmental Dental Abnormalities

Developmental abnormalities occur commonly in dogs and occasionally in cats. They can be caused by abnormal genetic coding or by damage to developing tissues. The necessity of treatment is based on whether the abnormality negatively impacts the health, function, or comfort of the patient. Radiographic evaluation of the extent of involvement helps the clinician to determine which abnormalities require immediate intervention, which might require treatment or monitoring, and which do not require any intervention at all.

## Abnormal Tooth Shape or Structure

Trauma to a deciduous tooth or inflammation from a fractured deciduous tooth can damage the enamel epithelium of the underlying developing permanent tooth, resulting in a focal area of enamel hypoplasia or hypomineralization (Figure 9-1). This is usually radiographically unremarkable, but a radiograph should be made to evaluate pulp health prior to restoration (Figure 9-2).

Generalized enamel dysplasia can be caused by systemic diseases (for example, viral infection such as distemper) during development and also by hereditary or nutritional factors. Radiographs should be made to determine whether the tooth root development was also affected (Figures 9-3 and 9-4).

Supernumerary roots most commonly affect maxillary third premolar teeth in both dogs and cats (Figure 9-5). Most are not associated with pathology and may be considered a variation of normal. It can be clinically significant if it is associated with periodontitis, and during extraction or endodontic treatment of the tooth.

Trauma to a deciduous tooth can also cause dislocation of the underlying permanent tooth bud. When one part of the developing tooth is repositioned relative to other parts, it can result in dilaceration of the tooth, a severe angular defect of the erupting tooth often occurring at the junction of the root to the crown. A deformed tooth may be unable to erupt (Figure 9-6).

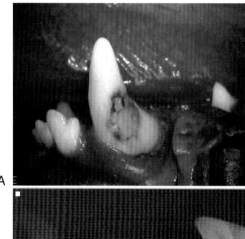

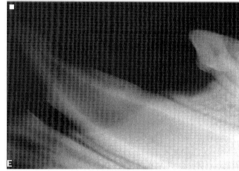

**FIGURE 9-1** Focal enamel defect ("Turner's tooth"). **A,** An area on the labial surface of a left mandibular canine tooth is missing the enamel layer and has poorly attached enamel on the periphery of the lesion. This area was close to the apex of the deciduous tooth during development. **B,** On the radiograph of the tooth in **A,** the crown is irregular with radiolucent surface defects and the pulp cavity appears normal.

Fusion of two tooth germs results in a single large tooth and one fewer tooth in the arch (Figure 9-7).

Gemination is the attempt of a single enamel organ to make two teeth. The result is a tooth with two crowns on one root (Figures 9-8 and 9-9). In single-rooted teeth, this cannot be differentiated from the fusion of the root of a normal tooth with that of a supernumerary tooth. In multirooted teeth,

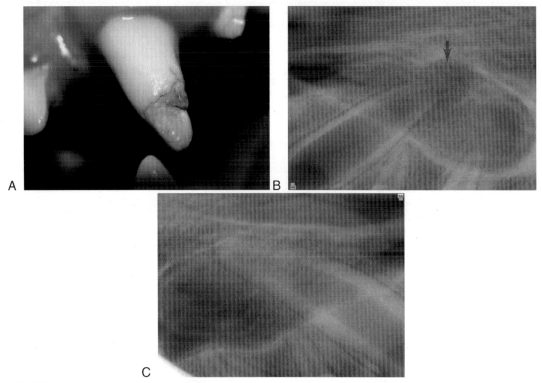

**FIGURE 9-2 Enamel-dentin lesion with endodontic involvement. A,** The coronal third of the canine tooth crown is deformed, is missing enamel, and has a defect extending into a groove in the dentin. **B,** On the radiograph of the tooth in **A,** there is a periapical lucency (*arrow*), indicating endodontic involvement. **C,** The contralateral tooth of the same patient has a narrower root canal space, indicating further maturation than the tooth in **B**.

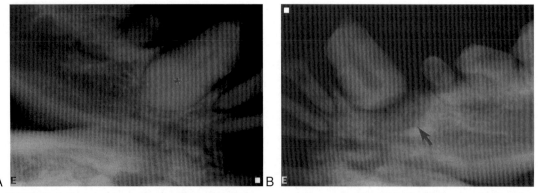

**FIGURE 9-3 Enamel and dentin dysplasia. A,** The root of the canine tooth (*asterisk*) is very short due to lack of development. **B,** On the contralateral tooth of the same patient a radiolucency (*arrow*) surrounds the shortened root, indicating loss of periodontal attachment. The wide root canal space is consistent with pulp necrosis.

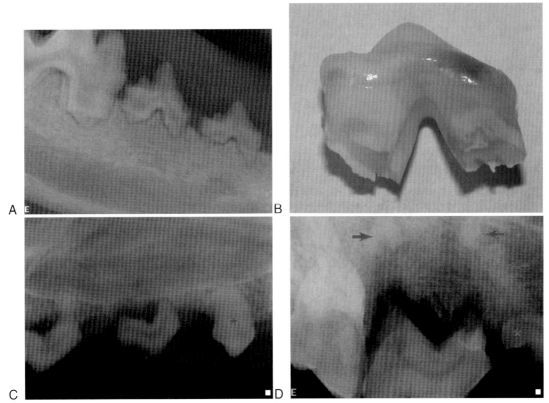

**FIGURE 9-4 Enamel and dentin dysplasia. A,** These mandibular premolar and molar teeth had enamel defects. The roots are very short and attenuated with narrow apices. The shape of these roots is characteristic of radicular dentin dysplasia in humans (also called type 1 dentin dysplasia, rootless teeth, type 1 dentinogenesis imperfecta), an autosomal dominant hereditary disturbance of dentin formation. However, in the human syndrome, the pulp cavity is generally attenuated or absent and the enamel is not affected. **B,** This tooth was extracted after becoming necrotic due to trauma during development. Its shape demonstrates early crown development prior to any root formation. Interruption of dentin formation or damage to the root-forming cells at this stage would result in teeth shaped like those in **A** and **C. C,** Radiographs indicate the timing of the insult by which roots are involved. In this patient, development was hindered after most of the root of the first premolar tooth (*asterisk*) was formed but before those of the second and third premolars were formed. **D,** Resorptive lesions can mimic roots affected by dentin dysplasia. However, residual root tips (*arrows*) of the resorbing maxillary fourth premolar tooth can be seen. The third premolar tooth (*asterisk*) also has evidence of root resorption.

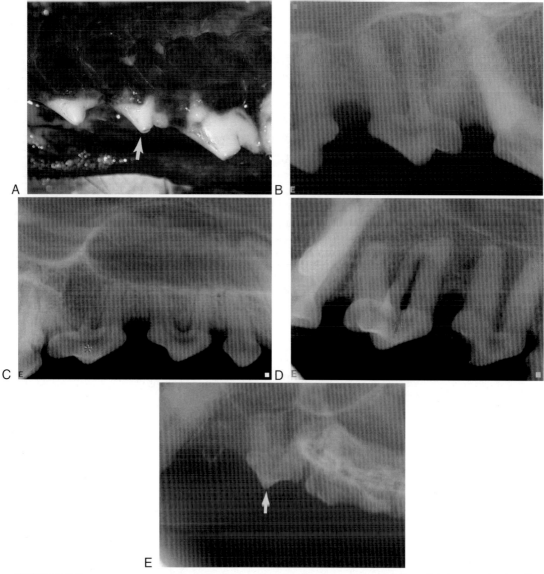

**FIGURE 9-5 Supernumerary root. A,** Palatal mirror image view of a maxillary third premolar tooth with a palatal root (*arrow*). **B,** Radiograph of the tooth in **A.** This tooth normally has two roots. **C,** Short supernumerary root on a third premolar tooth (*asterisk*). **D,** Long supernumerary root with vertical bone loss (*arrow*). **E,** Supernumerary root on a third premolar (*arrow*) of a cat.

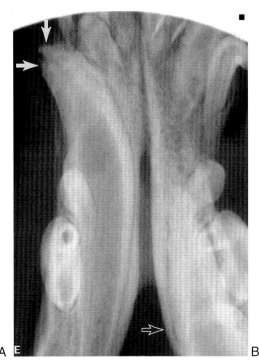
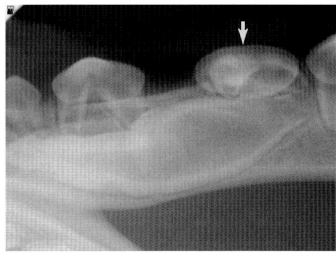

A   B

**FIGURE 9-6 Dilacerated unerupted tooth. A,** On a ventrodorsal radiograph, the right mandibular canine tooth is incompletely erupted and has defects of the enamel (*arrows*). The left canine tooth crown is adjacent to the first, second, and third premolar teeth. There is an angular defect where the crown meets the root (open arrow). **B,** The developing root extended caudally in the mandible, displacing the third premolar tooth (*arrow*).

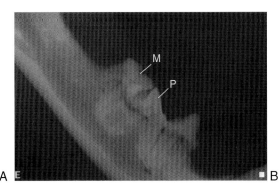
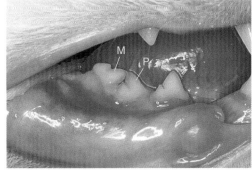

A   B

**FIGURE 9-7 Fusion of teeth in a cat. A,** The right mandibular fourth premolar tooth (P) and molar tooth (M) are fused, forming one large central shared root. **B,** The clinical appearance of fourth premolar and molar tooth fusion.

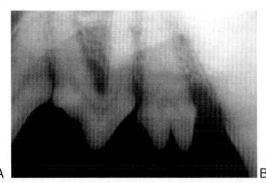
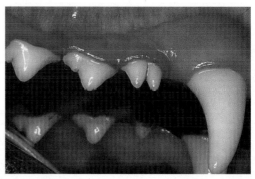

**FIGURE 9-8** **Gemination. A,** The right maxillary first premolar tooth has a singe root and the appearance of a bifid crown. **B,** Clinically, there are two crowns in close apposition to each other.

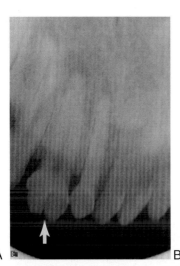
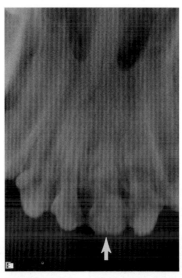
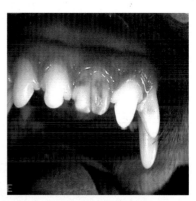

**FIGURE 9-9** **Gemination. A,** The right maxillary second incisor tooth (*arrow*) has a double crown and an abnormally wide root. The periapical lucency is rounder and more blunted than a normal chevron lucency, indicating endodontic involvement. **B,** On a radiograph of another patient, the coronal section of the root of the left maxillary first incisor tooth (*arrow*) is abnormal but the apical section appears more normal. **C,** The crown of the tooth in **B** is wide and discolored and has an asymmetric diagonal developmental groove. These findings are consistent with trauma during development that was followed by continued dentin and root development.

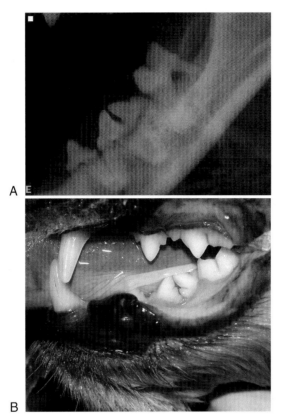

**FIGURE 9-10** **Fused supernumerary tooth in a cat. A,** There is a supernumerary left mandibular fourth premolar tooth positioned in the arch. It is fused with the other fourth premolar tooth similar to the premolar-molar fusion in Figure 9-7. **B,** There is an additional tooth in the quadrant.

fusion of supernumerary teeth is more apparent (Figure 9-10). When complete separation forms two teeth from one tooth germ, the result is a type of supernumerary tooth called "twinning" (Figure 9-11). Supernumerary mandibular fourth premolar tooth are commonly bilateral in cats.

Teeth affected by focal or localized microdontia (smaller size than normal) are often abnormally shaped (Figure 9-12). One form of this is a conical shaped tooth (Figure 9-12*A*), sometimes called a "peg tooth," in a tooth that normally has coronally divergent proximal surfaces.

Convergent roots (Figure 9-13) occur most commonly on mandibular first molar teeth in small-breed dogs. Affected teeth frequently develop endodontic disease. The clinical crowns of affected molar teeth often appear normal except for a developmental groove close to the mid-buccal gingival margin. Premolar teeth can also have convergent roots, sometimes with incomplete separation of the roots during development.

Dens in dente, or dens invaginatus, is an infolding of the developing tooth of varying severity that can result in periodontal problems and endodontic involvement (Figure 9-14).

Enamel pearls are deposits of enamel on the root (Figure 9-15) that sometimes have dentin involvement and rarely pulp as well. Because the periodontal ligament cannot attach to enamel, they may contribute to periodontitis.

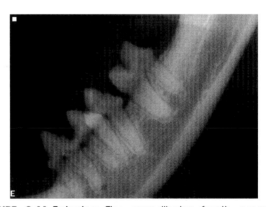

**FIGURE 9-11** **Twinning.** The mandibular fourth premolar tooth and supernumerary tooth are positioned side-by-side in the mandible, increasing the likelihood of crowding and occlusal interference. The superimposed roots cause increased radiopacity. The presence or extent of fusion cannot always be determined radiographically.

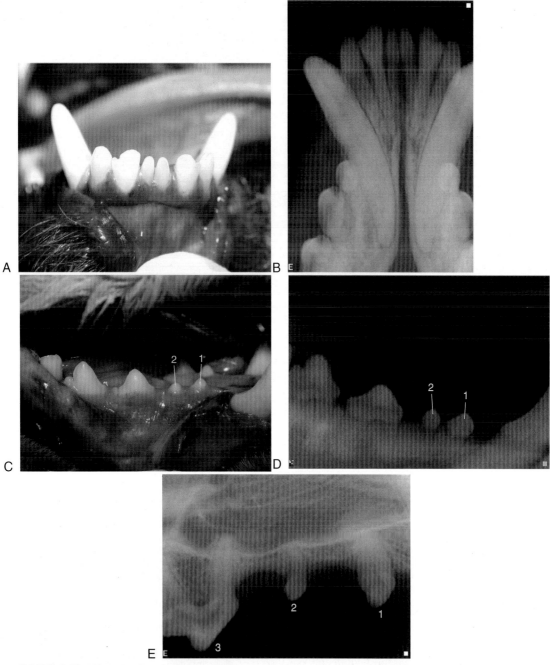

**FIGURE 9-12 Microdontia. A,** Both mandibular first incisor teeth are smaller than normal and have conical crowns (peg teeth). **B,** On a radiograph of the patient in **A,** the crowns of the first incisor teeth are small and there is alveolar bone loss around them. **C,** The right mandibular second premolar (2) is narrower and shorter than the first premolar (1). **D,** On a radiograph of the patient in **C,** the second premolar tooth has only one root instead of the normal two roots. **E,** The right maxillary second premolar tooth (2) is small and has only one root. The small size results in wide interproximal spaces between it and the first (1) and third (3) premolar teeth.

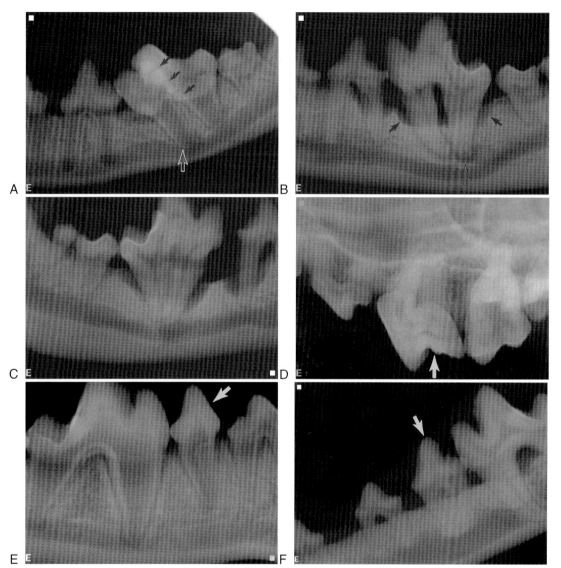

FIGURE 9-13 **Convergent roots. A,** The mesial root of the mandibular first molar tooth is positioned distal to the normal position (*open arrow*). The developmental groove and coronal displacement of the pulp floor (*arrows*) make an appearance similar to a dens-in-dente. **B,** A similar case in a more mature dog. There is alveolar bone loss (*arrows*) and a periapical lucency of endodontic origin (*open arrow*). **C,** An even more severe example of convergent roots. **D,** Convergent roots on a maxillary fourth premolar tooth (*arrow*). **E,** Convergent roots on a rotated mandibular fourth premolar (*arrow*). **F,** Convergent roots on a mandibular fourth premolar (*arrow*) with fusion of the root tips.

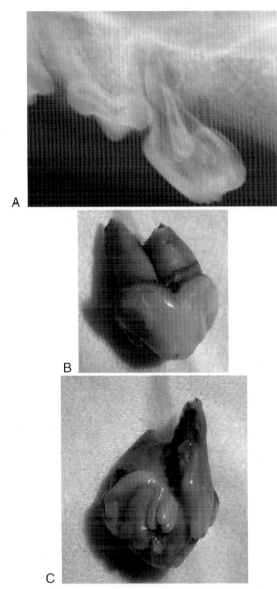

FIGURE 9-14 Dens in dente, or dens invaginatus, is an in-folding of the tooth prior to calcification. On a radiograph it appears like a tooth within a tooth, thus its name. **A,** Radiograph of a dens in dente maxillary premolar tooth on a dog. **B,** The extracted tooth appears only moderately deformed on the buccal surface. The roots are wide and calculus extends onto the root surface. **C,** The palatal surface is severely distorted. (*Photographs courtesy of Dr. Izumi Kitamura.*)

## Abnormal Tooth Number

Hypodontia, or missing teeth (Figure 9-16), can be genetic or can be the result of a disturbance during the early stages of tooth formation. Hypodontia usually presents no clinical problems for dogs and cats. Because dogs and cats do not experience mesial migration or drift, gaps in the dentition are less important.

Polyodontia (hyperdontia), or supernumerary teeth, are generally caused by a genetic abnormality. Incisor teeth and premolar teeth are the most commonly affected teeth,

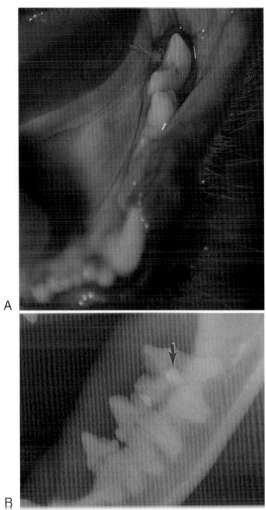

FIGURE 9-15 Enamel pearl. **A,** An enamel structure (*arrow*) protrudes through the lingual gingiva adjacent to the mandibular molar of a cat. **B,** On a radiograph of the patient in **A,** the enamel pearl is seen as a radiopacity in the mid-lingual cervical area of the molar tooth (*arrow*).

but molars and canines can also be affected. Supernumerary teeth in areas with minimal-to-no intercuspation and open contacts generally do not cause any problems. They do cause problems, however, when they result in crowding, diminished self-cleaning, or traumatic occlusion (Figure 9-17).

Supernumerary maxillary first premolar teeth in dogs (Figure 9-18) and second premolar teeth in cats are often clinically insignificant. They are sometimes supplemental teeth with the appearance of a normal tooth in a normal position in the arch. They are also sometimes abnormally shaped. Cats sometimes have supernumerary mandibular fourth premolars that can be complete twins, occupying the same position side-by-side in the mandible (see Figure 9-11). This condition is often bilateral. Either way, they are likely to cause problems due to traumatic contact with the maxillary dentition, crowding, and secondary periodontitis.

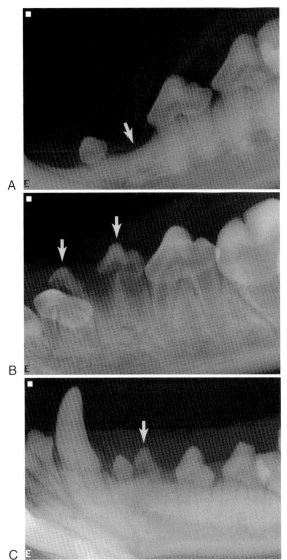

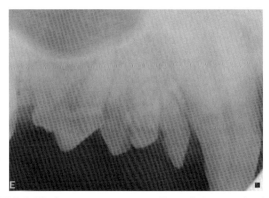

**FIGURE 9-17.** Supernumerary maxillary first premolar tooth with crowding.

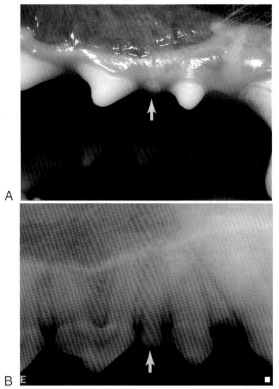

**FIGURE 9-16 Hypodontia.** The area of the congenitally missing mandibular second premolar tooth (*arrow*) is characterized by a uniform alveolar bone margin, no evidence of healing alveoli or previous roots, and a wide gap in the dentition where a permanent tooth should reside. **B,** The deciduous second and third premolar crowns (*arrows*) are present but there is no succedaneous permanent third premolar tooth. The deciduous tooth appears ready to exfoliate. **C,** On this radiograph of an older dog. The deciduous mandibular second premolar tooth (*arrow*) also has no permanent tooth replacement but has solid roots. Deciduous teeth sometimes remain in function for many years.

**FIGURE 9-18 Supernumerary maxillary first premolar tooth** (*arrow*) **without crowding. A,** Clinical picture. **B,** Radiograph.

## Abnormal Position or Eruption

In addition to interference with eruption caused by malformation as discussed earlier, teeth can fail to erupt or erupt in abnormal positions from other causes.

Persistent deciduous teeth are generally somehow related to lack of close proximity of their roots to the eruption pathway of the successional permanent teeth. This physical relationship is one important component of deciduous tooth exfoliation (see Chapter 2). If either the deciduous or permanent tooth is malpositioned (usually a genetic trait), or if there is no permanent successor (also usually genetic), the deciduous tooth may not exfoliate normally. Hormonal or metabolic problems can also cause this.

Delayed eruption of permanent teeth is common in some breeds. Failure to properly erupt can also be genetic. Tissue covering a tooth that is nearly in an erupted position should be excised to facilitate the final eruptive stages. A preoperative radiograph may be helpful to anticipate the presence of bone that also must be removed (Figure 9-19).

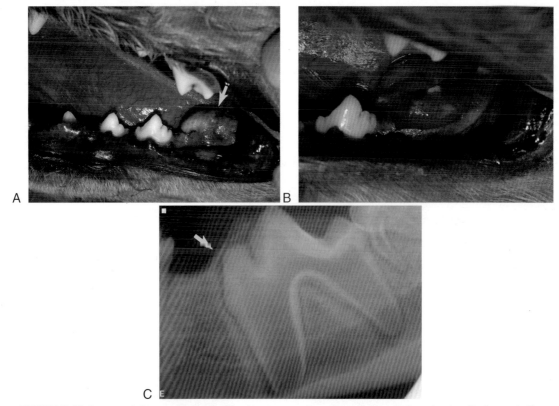

**FIGURE 9-19 Incomplete eruption. A,** Gingiva covers the mandibular first molar tooth (*arrow*). The gingival contour suggests near-normal tooth position. **B,** The soft tissue has been incised and is lifted to reveal the underlying bony collar that also must be removed. **C,** On a radiograph of the tooth in **A** and **B**, the mesial aspect is incompletely erupted with significant reserve crown and overlying bony tissue (*arrow*). The radiograph provides information about what to expect during operculectomy surgery.

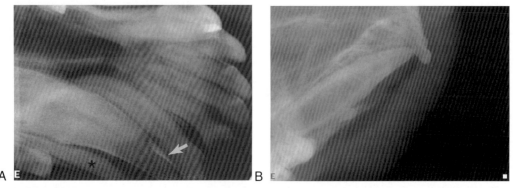

**FIGURE 9-20 Lance projection canine teeth. A,** The mesioverted right maxillary canine tooth of a dog is touching the third incisor tooth, eliminating the normal diastema (*arrow*) in which the mandibular canine tooth ordinarily rests. The deciduous canine tooth persists (*asterisk*). **B,** A lance projection canine tooth in a cat.

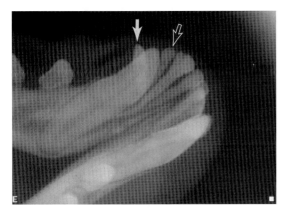

**FIGURE 9-21** Mesioverted mandibular canine tooth with impaction against the incisor teeth. The permanent third incisor tooth (*arrow*) is displaced distally by the canine tooth. The deciduous third incisor tooth (*open arrow*) is persistent.

Malposed permanent teeth can be genetic, such as mesioversion/lance projection of canine teeth (Figure 9-20) commonly seen in Shelties and Dachshunds and occasionally in other breeds. It can also be the result of trauma to a deciduous tooth that dislocated the permanent tooth bud. The developing bud is very easily moved because there is no periodontal ligament in the early stage. Teeth that erupt in an abnormal position or angle can cause traumatic occlusion, can impact against other structures in the same arch (Figure 9-21), and can result in crowding with predisposition to periodontitis.

## SUGGESTED READINGS

Avery JK (ed): *Oral development and histology,* New York, 1994, Thieme.

Gibilesco JA: *Stafne's Oral radiographic diagnosis,* Philadelphia, 1985, WB Saunders.

Neville BW, Damm DD, White DK, Waldron CA: *Color atlas of clinical oral pathology,* Philadelphia, 1991, Lea and Febiger.

Regezi JA, Sciubba J: *Oral pathology, clinical-pathologic correlations,* ed 2, Philadelphia, 1993, WB Saunders.

Wiggs RB, Lobprise HB: *Veterinary dentistry principles and practice,* Philadelphia, 1997, Lippincott–Raven.

Zwemer TJ: *Boucher's Clinical dental terminology, a glossary of accepted terms in all disciplines of dentistry,* ed 4, St. Louis, 1993, Mosby–Year Book.

# CHAPTER 10

# Trauma

Traumatic injuries to the face, head, and teeth occur in dogs and cats for many reasons, including motor vehicle accidents, accidental striking injuries (i.e., baseball bat, tennis racket, golf club), fighting with another animal, falling, and running into objects, as well as self-inflicted trauma from chewing and biting on hard or abrasive objects. Injuries may involve the teeth, jaws, or bones of the head including the bones of the temporomandibular joint (TMJ)

Radiographic evaluation of the patient's head injuries is done after complete patient evaluation and stabilization. Dental radiographs are made to assess traumatic injuries to the teeth, alveolar bone, mandible, maxilla, and TMJ. Depending on the injuries, skull radiographs and computed tomography scans may be recommended for complete evaluation of all injuries.

Patients with obvious traumatic injuries to their teeth frequently have no known history of trauma. An owner may notice that a tooth is missing or fractured and have no idea how it happened. When a tooth is missing without a known history of extraction, a dental radiograph is recommended. Traumatic injuries often lead to root fractures, loss of tooth crown, and retention of tooth root. Radiographs are made to identify persistent roots and any associated pathology (Figure 10-1, *A*). A crown fracture that exposes the pulp chamber will result in endodontic disease. When this occurs, the extent of pathology should be evaluated with a dental radiograph (Figure 10-1, *B*).

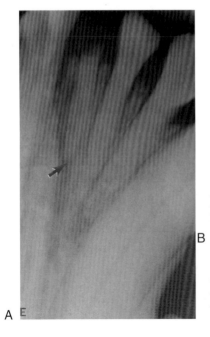
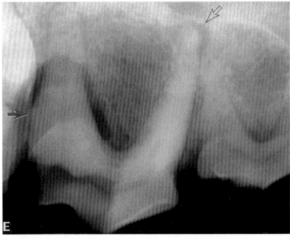

**FIGURE 10-1 A,** Persistent root and periapical lucency (*arrow*) of a fractured left mandibular first incisor in a dog with no known dental trauma. **B,** Fractured right maxillary fourth premolar with pulp chamber exposure, periodontal bone loss (*arrow*), and radiographic evidence of a periapical abscess (widening of the periodontal ligament space, loss of the radiopaque lamina dura, and radiolucency at apex) (*open arrow*).

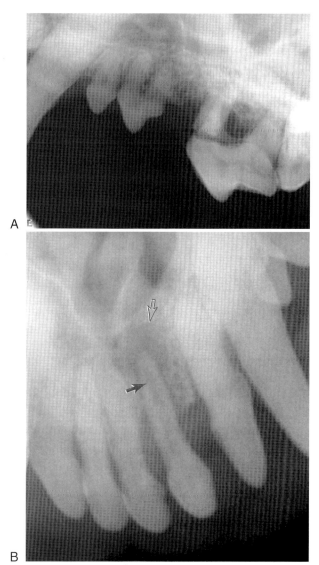

A

B

**FIGURE 10-2 A,** Fractured left maxillary fourth premolar in a Chihuahua with no known history of trauma. **B,** On this radiograph of a discolored maxillary first incisor, there is a wide root canal (*arrow*) and periapical lucency (*open arrow*), indicating pulp necrosis and chronic inflammation.

Traumatic tooth injuries are frequently noted for the first time when an oral examination is done as part of a physical examination or when a patient is under general anesthesia for performing periodontal treatment (Figure 10-2, *A*). Blunt trauma may result in damage to the pulp without fracturing the tooth. A dental radiograph should be made of any tooth that is discolored from pulp hemorrhage (Figure 10-2, *B*).

Root fractures with or without concurrent crown fractures occur secondary to trauma and affect the prognosis and treatment of the tooth (Figure 10-3).

Self-inflicted trauma to teeth occurs from chewing on a variety of inappropriate materials and objects that may cause soft-tissue trauma and excessive wear, concussive trauma, fracture, or luxation of teeth (Figures 10-4 through 10-8).

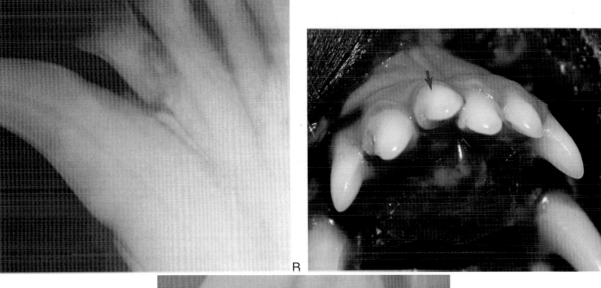

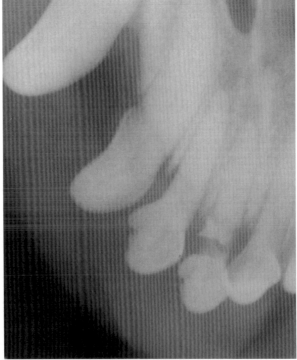

**FIGURE 10-3 A,** Crown and root fractures of the right mandibular third incisor. **B,** The deviated maxillary right first incisor (*arrow*) had increased mobility. **C,** Crown-root fracture of incisor shown in **B.**

Dogs and cats that fight with each other may receive trauma from bites, blunt force, or pulling forces (i.e., tooth caught in collar) (Figures 10.9 through 10.11).

Maxillofacial and mandibular fractures may result in traumatic injuries to the teeth as well as the bone (Figures 10-12 and 10-13).

Dogs and cats that are struck by motor vehicles often receive significant head trauma and multiple fractures (Figures 10-14 through 10-16).

Iatrogenic trauma may occur when performing an extraction (i.e., fractured mandible) or when placing pins to stabilize a fracture (Figure 10-17).

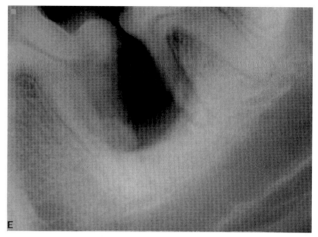

**FIGURE 10-4** Severe bone loss between the left mandibular first and second molar in a dog that had impacted grass and wood between the teeth.

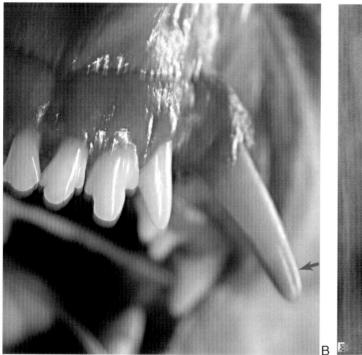

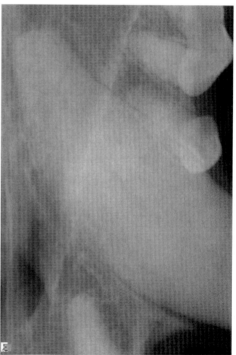

**FIGURE 10-5 A,** Laterally deviated maxillary left canine tooth with purple discoloration of the crown (*arrow*) in a dog with a history of chasing cars and chewing on tires. This can be a result of intraalveolar root fracture or of tooth luxation. **B,** On a radiograph of the deviated tooth in **A,** there is no evidence of root fracture.

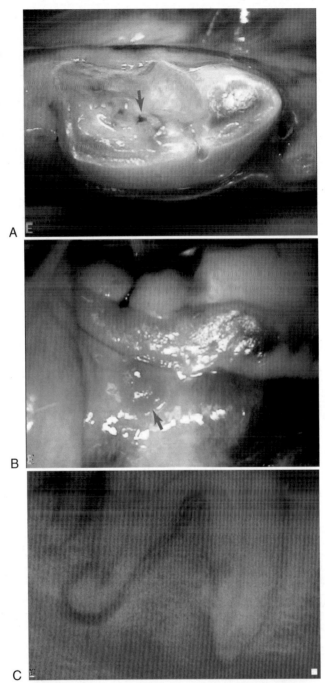

**FIGURE 10-6 A,** Chronic wear of right lower first molar with focal dark areas (*arrow*) of possible pulp exposure. **B,** Focal erythematous area (*arrow*) of alveolar mucosa adjacent to distal root of first molar in **A**. **C,** Periapical lucency (*arrow*) secondary to chronic endodontic disease.

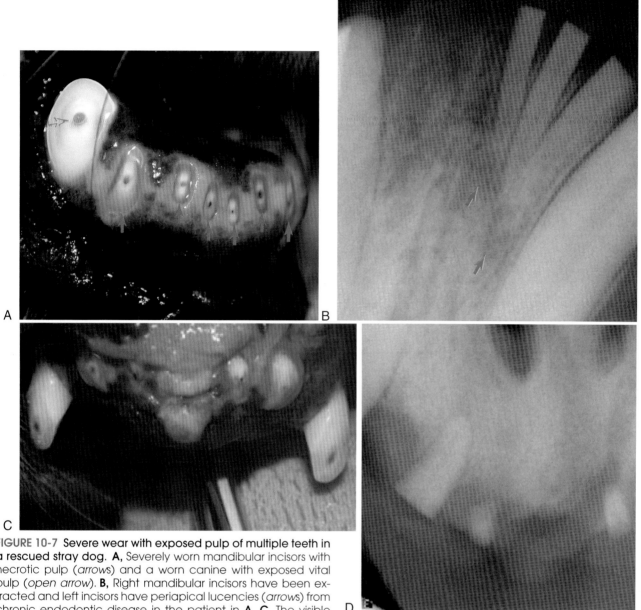

**FIGURE 10-7** Severe wear with exposed pulp of multiple teeth in a rescued stray dog. **A,** Severely worn mandibular incisors with necrotic pulp (*arrows*) and a worn canine with exposed vital pulp (*open arrow*). **B,** Right mandibular incisors have been extracted and left incisors have periapical lucencies (*arrows*) from chronic endodontic disease in the patient in **A. C,** The visible incisors and canine teeth are severely worn into the pulp chambers. **D,** Severe bone loss surrounding the roots of the left and right maxillary second incisors in the patient in **C.**

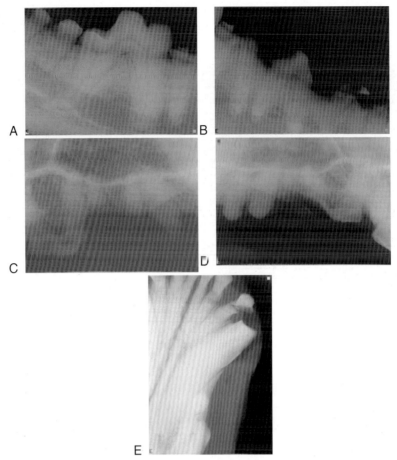

**FIGURE 10-8** Radiographs of traumatic damage to multiple teeth in a dog with separation anxiety that was placed in a crate for 30 minutes. **A,** Crown fracture of mandibular right second molar and fourth premolar. **B,** Crown fractures of right mandibular second and fourth premolars. **C,** Missing crown with retained roots of the right maxillary second premolar. **D,** Crown fracture of maxillary left second premolar and supernumerary first premolar. **E,** Crown fracture of left mandibular canine tooth and crown-root fractures of left mandibular third and second incisors.

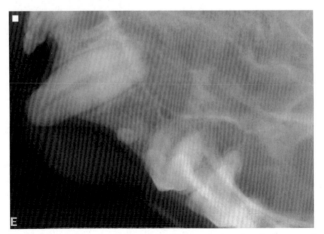

**FIGURE 10-9** Fractured left maxillary canine tooth in a cat secondary to trauma from fighting with another cat.

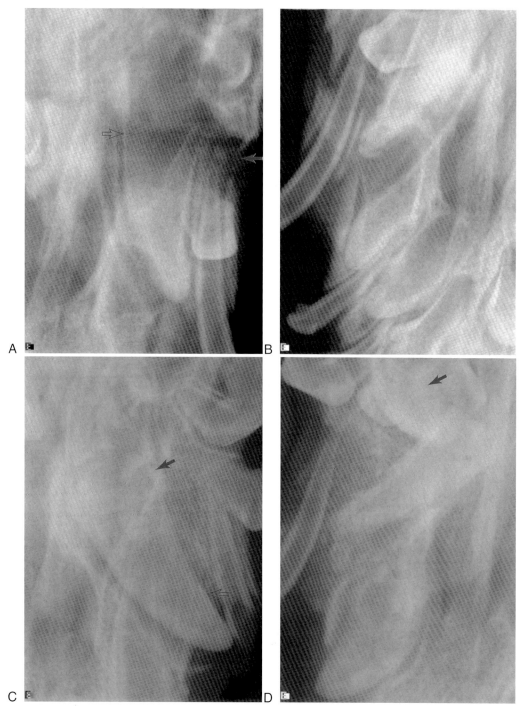

**FIGURE 10-10** Radiographs of an 11-week-old puppy with acute trauma from a dog bite (**A, B**) and 11 weeks later (**C, D**). **A,** Fractured maxillary bone (*arrows*) in area of developing left permanent canine tooth, **B,** Fractured right maxillary bone. **C,** Left permanent canine crown (*open arrow*) appears normal; root development is abnormal (*arrow*). **D,** Abnormal development of right permanent canine tooth (*arrow*).

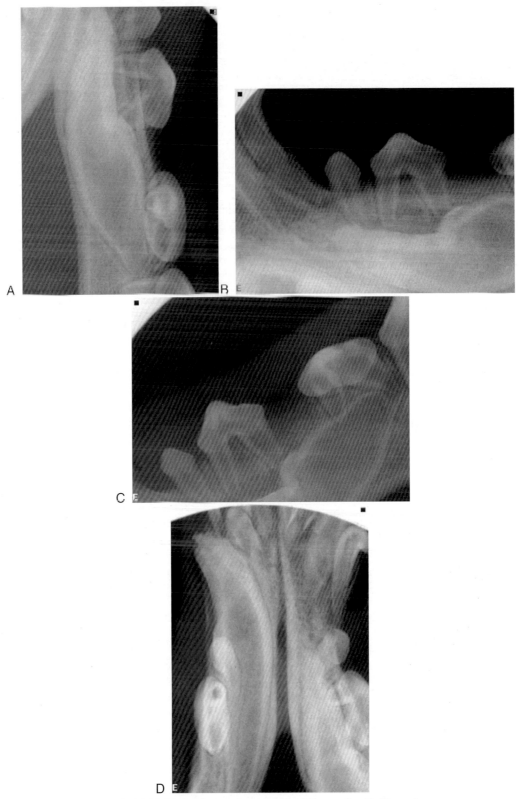

**FIGURE 10-11** Radiographs made at 7½ months (**A-D**) and 11 months (**E, F**) of age in a dog that was bitten in the face by another dog at 12 weeks of age. **A-C,** Embedded left mandibular canine tooth. **D,** Unerupted right lower canine tooth with coronal enamel defect.

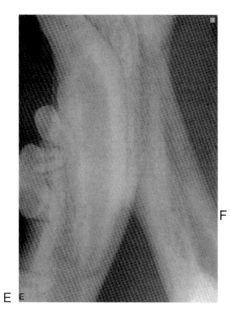

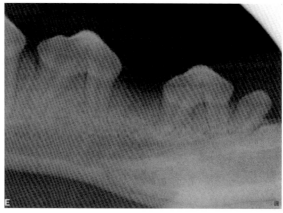

FIGURE 10-11, cont'd **E, F,** Continued development of unerupted right lower canine tooth.

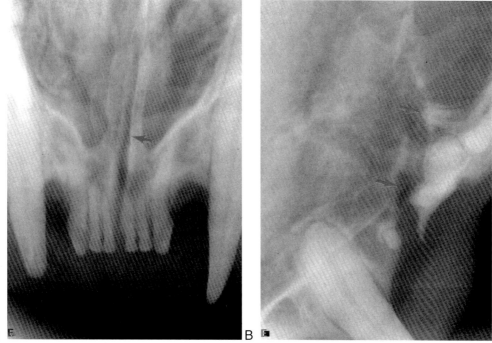

FIGURE 10-12 Radiographs made of a cat with head trauma of unknown cause. **A,** Separation of median palatal suture (*arrow*). **B,** Fracture of left maxillary bone with potential trauma to the adjacent second and third premolars (*arrows*).

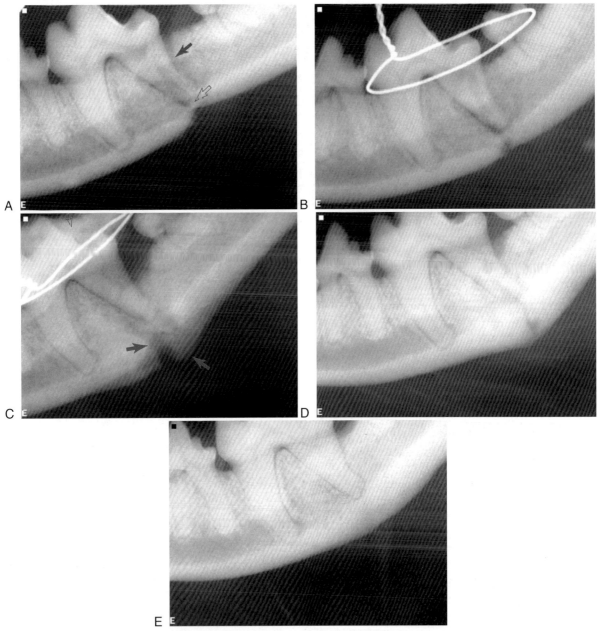

**FIGURE 10-13** Radiographs made of an adult Lhasa Apso with a fractured left mandible. **A,** The fracture line extends through the distal alveolar bone (*arrow*) and periapical area (*open arrow*) of the distal root of the first molar. **B,** Radiograph made to evaluate the apposition of the fractured segments after stabilization with interdental wiring. **C,** Interfragmentary callus formation (*arrows*) is present at 4 weeks after initial fracture stabilization. Acrylic composite material (*open arrow*) and wire were not removed. **D,** Bridging callus formation has occurred stabilizing the fracture at 10 weeks postfracture stabilization and the wire and acrylic material were removed. **E,** Radiographs were made at 6 months postrepair to evaluate the first molar for endodontic problems. The ventral cortex of the mandible has decreased in thickness as remodeling has occurred and the periodontal ligament spaces of the first molar appear normal in width.

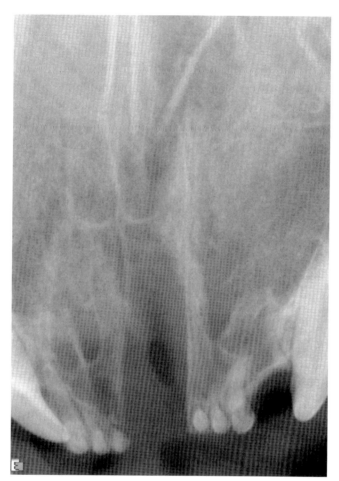

FIGURE 10-14 Fractured and separated maxillary bones in a cat with severe head trauma.

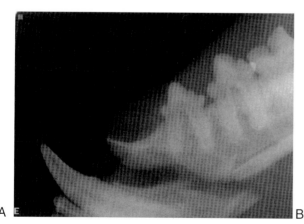

A

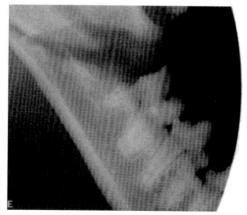

B

FIGURE 10-15 Radiographs of a cat with severe head trauma. **A,** Oblique fracture of the rostral left mandible. **B,** Oblique fracture of distal right mandible.

*Continued.*

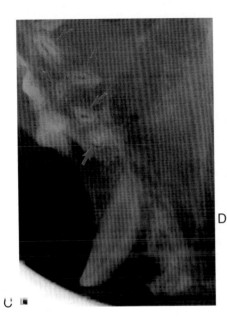

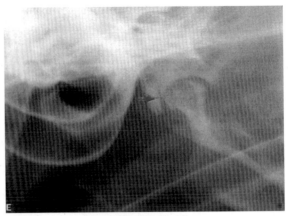

FIGURE 10-15, cont'd **C,** Maxillary and premolar crown fractures separating the third and fourth premolar crowns from the roots (*arrows*). **D,** Fracture of right mandibular fossa (*arrow*) with minimal displacement.

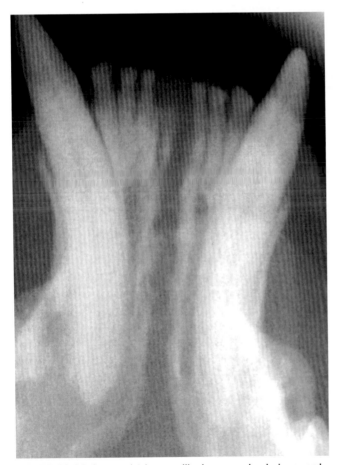

FIGURE 10-16 Separated mandibular symphysis in a cat with head trauma.

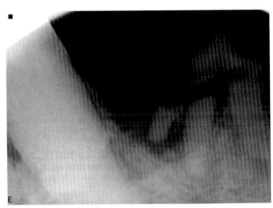

FIGURE 10-17 Iatrogenic trauma caused by pins placed to stabilize a mandibular fracture.

## SUGGESTED READING

Verstraete FJM: Maxillofacial fractures, In Slatter D, editor: *Textbook of small animal surgery*, Philadelphia, 2003, W.B. Saunders, pp 2190-2207.

# CHAPTER 11

# Miscellaneous Conditions

## Osteomyelitis

Osteomyelitis in the jaws most commonly arises from dental infections and persistent infected roots (Figure 11-1). Infection that has spread into the bone is more difficult to resolve due to the establishment of a bacterial biofilm with its inherent protective mechanisms. Acute osteomyelitis may exhibit no radiographic abnormalities. Established infection usually appears as an area of relative radiolucency with poorly defined margins (see Chapter 6).

Sclerosing osteomyelitis (condensing osteitis, bony scar, sclerotic bone, focal periapical osteopetrosis) is an inflammatory condition believed to be a local bony reaction to a low-grade inflammatory stimulus or to bacteria of low virulence. Focal sclerosing osteitis appears radiographically as an opacity at, or in the vicinity of, the apex or lateral canal of a tooth that has had a long-lasting pulpitis (Figure 11-2). The periodontal ligament and root remain distinct from the opacity. The focal lesion may be uniformly opaque, may be peripherally lucent with an opaque center, or may be composed of confluent or lobulated opaque masses. The radiographic appearance can be similar to that of periapical cemental dysplasia, complex odontoma, osteoblastoma, and hypercementosis.

The diffuse form of sclerosing osteomyelitis affects a larger area of the jaw. Early in the course, there are lucent zones in association with sclerotic masses (Figure 11-3). In advanced stages, it is characterized by a generalized increased opacity (Figure 11-4).

## Opacities Not Caused by Inflammation or Infection

Osteosclerosis can also occur in the absence of inflammation or infection (Figure 11-5). A common site in humans is the septal bone between premolar teeth. One theory suggests the cause is persistent fragments of primary teeth that become encapsulated by cementum.

Periapical cemental dysplasia (also called cementoma, cementifying fibroma, ossifying fibroma, enostosis, and periapical ossifying dysplasia) has been classified as a mesenchymal tumor but also as a reaction to an unknown factor, and its etiology is unsure. The stage 1 lesion of periapical cemental dysplasia is a periapical lucency that appears radiographically similar to a lesion of endodontic origin but is associated with a tooth with a healthy pulp. In the stage 2 lesion, the central part of the lesion is filled with mineralized material (Figure 11-6). Stage 3 lesions become completely opaque. They tend to be asymptomatic and usually do not require any intervention.

Persistent root fragments appear as radiopacities that are identifiable by their characteristic shape and a surrounding periodontal ligament or inflammatory lesion. If there is any evidence of lucency or increased opacity around the fragment, it should be surgically removed. However, intervention may not be necessary if the root fragment is not associated with any radiolucency or bony changes (Figure 11-7). In this case, the client should be advised of the need to monitor with future radiographs.

Subgingival calculus deposits appear as radiopacities associated with a tooth root (Figure 11-8). They are usually surrounded by a region of radiolucency caused by periodontitis and inflammation.

Hypercementosis (cemental dysplasia) occurs when excess cementum is formed on the root, most commonly affecting the apical third (Figure 11-9). It is of no clinical importance unless there is an associated lucency or other evidence of pulp pathosis. The only inherent significance is to not extract the affected tooth thinking it is a problem, and if an affected tooth must be extracted for unrelated reasons, the club-like contour can complicate the extraction.

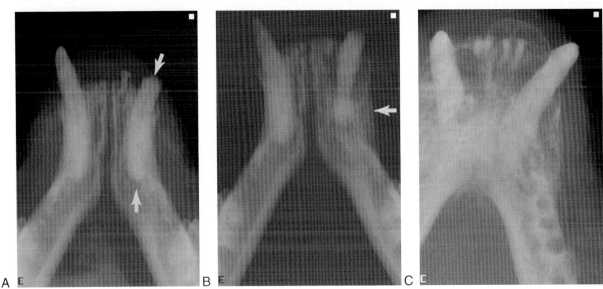

**FIGURE 11-1** Osteomyelitis in cats. **A,** Fractured mandibular left canine tooth with pulp exposure (*arrow*). The periapical area is characterized by a periapical lucency of endodontic origin (*open arrow*) (see Chapter 6). The roots of multiple incisor teeth persist. **B,** The patient in **A** was not treated and returned 2 years later. The canine root tip is displaced coronally as the tooth is supererupted (a misnomer in carnivore dentition). The coronal periodontal ligament is widened due to marginal alveolar expansion, and there is periosteal reaction and bone deposition on the labial aspect of the left mandible (*arrow*). These are all signs of localized osteomyelitis. **C,** Osteomyelitis secondary to periodontitis. The considerable bony reaction and enlargement give the radiographic appearance of a neoplastic process.

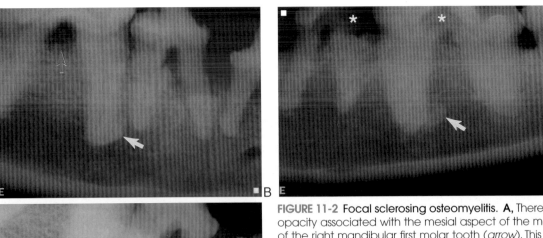

**FIGURE 11-2** Focal sclerosing osteomyelitis. **A,** There is a radiopacity associated with the mesial aspect of the mesial root of the right mandibular first molar tooth (*arrow*). This is likely a site of a lateral or apical canal. There is evidence of severe periodontitis and loss of alveolar marginal bone that has exposed the dentin and furcation area (*open arrow*), providing bacteria with potential access to the pulp through a furcal canal. **B,** A similar radiopacity on the distal aspect of the mesial root of a left mandibular first molar tooth (*arrow*). Tooth resorptions on the fourth premolar and first molar teeth appear as radiolucencies (*asterisks*). **C,** In this case, the sclerotic bone is not directly associated with the root tips (*arrows*).

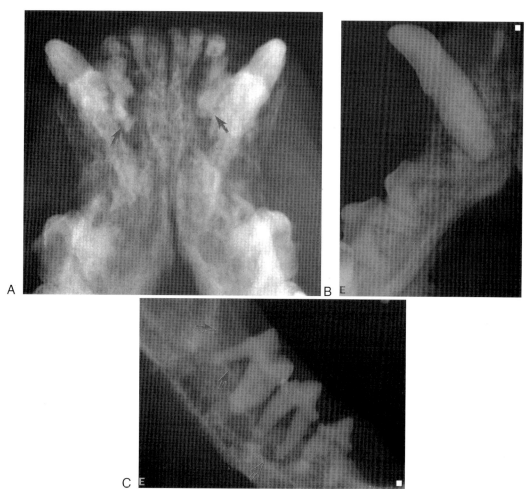

**FIGURE 11-3 Osteomyelitis secondary to periodontal disease. A,** The rostral mandibles of this cat are characterized by a generalized mottled appearance caused by areas of bone destruction and areas of unaffected or reactive bone. There are also significant subgingival calculus deposits (*arrows*) that contribute to the irregular opacity. The canine teeth roots have multiple tooth resorptions. **B,** Loss of trabeculation and a mottled appearance of the bone of the rostral mandible of a dog are evidence of osteomyelitis. **C,** The mandible of this cat has radiographic evidence of severe periodontitis (*arrows*), secondary endodontic involvement with periapical lucencies (*open arrow*), and a generalized mottled appearance with diffuse sclerosing osteomyelitis.

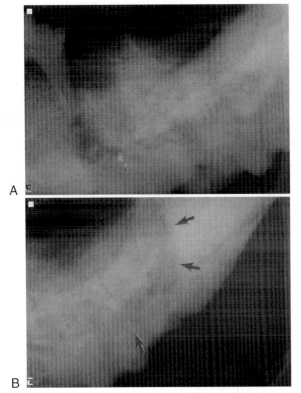

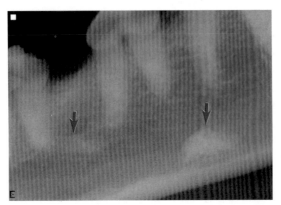

**FIGURE 11-4 Diffuse condensing osteomyelitis in a dog.**
**A,** The mandible from a dog characterized by generalized increased opacity. The molar teeth are missing. This patient had osteomyelitis, from which *Klebsiella, Proteus,* and *Escherichia coli* were isolated. **B,** Farther caudal on the mandible is a bony sequestrum visible radiographically as an area of increased radiopacity within a region of radiolucency (*arrows*).

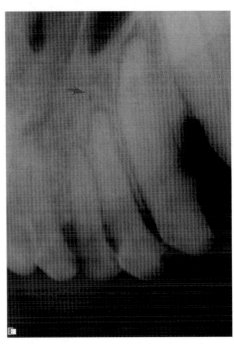

**FIGURE 11-6 Periapical cemental dysplasia (cementoma).**
In the stage 2 lesion, the central area of periapical lucency becomes radiopaque (*arrow*).

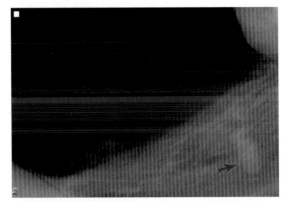

**FIGURE 11-7 The premolar teeth are missing.** There is a persistent root fragment (*arrow*). The alveolus appears to be healing and the periodontal ligament has established itself on the coronal surface.

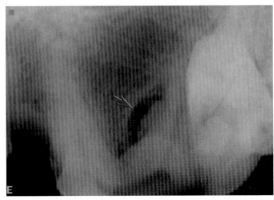

**FIGURE 11-5 Osteosclerosis.** Opacities in the mandible in the absence of endodontic disease or other identifiable pathology (*arrows*).

**FIGURE 11-8 Subgingival calculus deposit (*arrow*).**

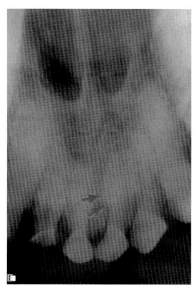

**FIGURE 11-9** Hypercementosis (cemental dysplasia). The apical halves of the roots of the maxillary incisor teeth are enlarged from increased cementum. The periodontal ligament follows the outer contour of the excess cementum (*arrows*).

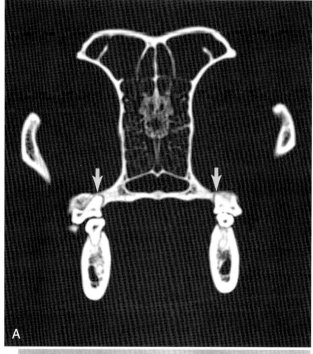

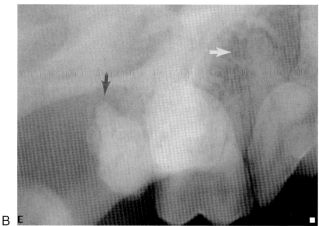

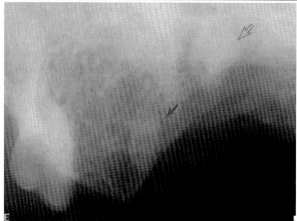

## Orbital Cellulitis

Inflammation of the orbital tissues can be caused by penetration of a foreign body from the oral cavity into the retromolar tissues or by extension of dental infections. The inflammation can progress to become a retrobulbar abscess. Clinical signs include proptosis, nictitans protrusion, inability to retropulse the globe, and severe pain on opening the mouth caused by pressure from the ramus of the mandible on the orbital contents. The roots most likely to result in orbital cellulitis are the distal roots of both molars and the palatal root of the first molar. These roots extend within millimeters of the dorsal bone of the maxillary tuberosity that forms the floor of the orbit behind the pterygopalatine fossa. This bone is perforated by foramina leading to their alveoli (Figure 11-10, *A* and *B*). It is also possible for the palatal root of the maxillary

**FIGURE 11-10** Orbital cellulitis. **A,** On the CT scan image, the distal and palatal roots of the maxillary first molar tooth (*arrows*) are very close to the orbital spaces. **B,** This patient had a retrobulbar abscess. On the radiograph, there is a large periapical lucency around the palatal root of the second molar tooth (*arrow*). It is difficult to discern in this area, but the caudal aspect of the alveolar process should encompass the palatal root. There is also periapical lucency affecting the distal root of the fourth premolar tooth (*open arrowhead*). **C,** This patient developed an acute orbital cellulitis 4 years after extraction of the fourth premolar and first molar teeth. Fragments of the mesiobuccal root of the first molar tooth (*arrow*) and the palatal root of the fourth premolar tooth (*open arrow*) persist. There was a large nasoalveolar defect connecting the infected palatal root to the nasal cavity, and the entire maxillary recess and caudal nasal cavity were filled with profuse necrotic and mucopurulent material.

fourth premolar tooth to extend to the orbit through a canal that connects the maxillary recess to the sphenopalatine foramen (Figure 11-10, *C*).

## Malocclusion

Oral radiographs can help determine whether teeth are missing or uncrupted (see Chapter 2, deciduous teeth). Interceptive orthodontic treatment can include extraction of deciduous teeth in young animals. Preoperative radiographs should be made to verify the presence of a successional permanent tooth and to confirm its location (Figure 11-11).

Traumatic contact from malocclusion can damage the opposing soft and hard tissues if not corrected early. It can also interfere with the normal eruptive processes of the con-

tacting teeth. Canine teeth that encounter an obstruction appear shorter due to incomplete eruption with an increased amount of reserved crown, and the root apex migrates caudally in the mandible as the root develops (Figure 11-12).

## Additional Findings

Radiographs are not necessary for the diagnosis of oronasal fistulation caused by periodontitis, but they can provide additional information about the degree of bone loss (Figure 11-13).

Caries is a bacterial infection that can infect the pulp. A radiograph should always be made prior to caries removal and tooth restoration to determine if endodontic treatment also needs to be performed (Figure 11-14).

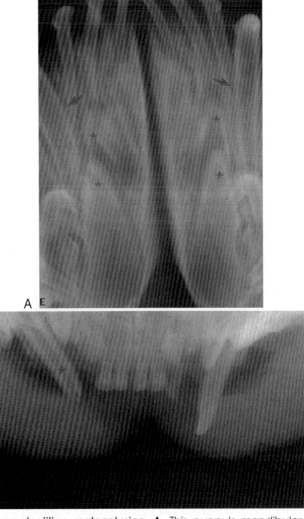

**FIGURE 11-11 Deciduous dentition malocclusion. A,** This puppy's mandibular deciduous canine teeth were impaling the palatal tissues. The location of the developing permanent canine and third incisor teeth (*asterisks*) places them at risk during extraction of the deciduous canines (*arrows*). **B,** Malocclusion in a kitten in the mixed dentition stage. The right maxillary deciduous canine tooth (*asterisk*) is palatoverted.

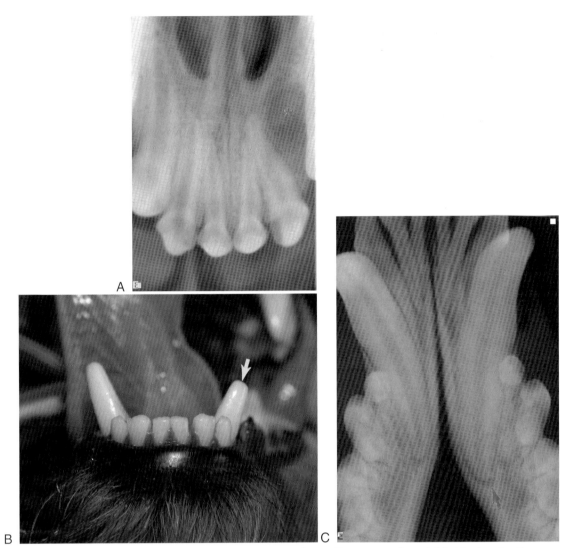

**FIGURE 11-12 Malocclusion. A,** The roots of the left maxillary second and third incisor teeth are displaced and separated by a lucency(*asterisk*). This is a defect in the palatal bone caused by trauma from the malpositioned mandibular canine tooth. **B,** This dog's left mandibular canine tooth (*arrow*) is incompletely erupted compared with the right one. **C,** The root apex of the left canine tooth is displaced caudally in the mandible (*arrow*), and the tooth is projected at a different angle from the right canine tooth.

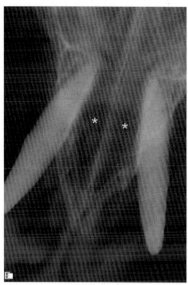

**FIGURE 11-13 Oronasal fistula.** The rostral maxillary region is characterized by extensive loss of both alveolar bone and palatal bone (*asterisks*).

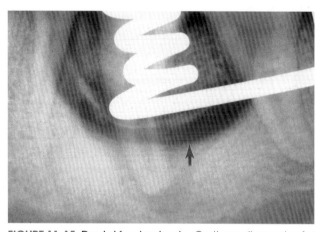

**FIGURE 11-15 Dental foreign body.** On the radiograph of a left mandibular first molar tooth of a dog, the coiled radiolucency is the metal spring of a clothespin that had clasped onto the tooth months earlier. The subjacent bone has developed a bony sequestrum separated from the vital bone by a radiolucent zone (*arrow*).

Radiographic evaluation of chronic injuries and foreign bodies help to evaluate the extent of bone involvement and can identify radiopaque foreign bodies (Figure 11-15).

Radiographs often only provide a list of possibilities and not the definitive diagnosis. They can hint at the active versus quiet nature of a lesion and whether immediate intervention, biopsy, or other additional diagnostic tests are urgent (Figure 11-16).

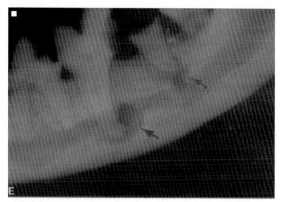

**FIGURE 11-14 Dental caries.** There is a large radiolucency of the crown of the left mandibular first molar tooth, and both roots are associated with periapical lucencies of endodontic origin (*arrows*). The distal root is exfoliating.

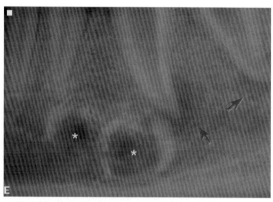

**FIGURE 11-16 Atypical manifestation of a radicular cyst or granuloma of endodontic origin.** The lesions are characterized by a central lucency (*asterisks*) surrounded by a discrete opacity. Radiographically, these have the same appearance as a calcifying odontogenic cyst, an ameloblastoma, a giant cell tumor, or a keratocyst. Differentiating between them requires histopathological evaluation. The root canal spaces of the first molar tooth are comparatively wider than those of adjacent teeth, indicating arrested maturation and pulp necrosis. There are periapical lucencies (*arrows*) around both roots consistent with rarefying osteitis.

## SUGGESTED READINGS

Neville BW, Damm DD, White DK, Waldron CA: *Color atlas of clinical oral pathology,* Philadelphia, 1991, Lea and Febiger.

Regezi JA, Sciubba J: *Oral pathology, clinical-pathologic correlations,* ed 2, Philadelphia, 1993, WB Saunders.

Slatter D, Basher T: Orbit. In Slatter D, editor: *Textbook of small animal surgery,* ed 3, Philadelphia, 2002, WB Saunders.

Wiggs RB, Lobprise HB: *Veterinary dentistry principles and practice,* Philadelphia, 1997, Lippincott–Raven.

# Technique

Poor-quality radiographs can contribute to inaccurate or missed diagnoses. Accurate and complete radiographic interpretation begins with high-quality radiographs. The first requirement for obtaining good radiographs is to have the correct radiographic equipment in good functional condition (see Chapter 13), the necessary supplies to develop the films, and the ability to use the equipment and supplies properly. Another important element is proper positioning. This chapter will discuss conventional dental radiography using dental x-ray film. Digital radiography will be considered in Chapter 13.

## Film

Dental film is available in a range of sensitivities, referred to as "film speeds," from A through F. The A speed film is the least sensitive, and F speed is the most sensitive. The sensitivity of the film determines the required exposure time; faster-speed (higher-sensitivity) film requires less radiation to expose (blacken) the film. Film sensitivity is increased by using larger silver halide crystals in the emulsion. As a result, E and F speed films produce images with a slightly lower image quality in the same manner that larger and fewer pixels decrease the image quality of digital camera images. The decreased image quality only becomes significant when viewed using magnification. D speed and E speed are commonly used. One popular film is E speed when hand processed and F speed when developed in an automatic processor (Kodak Insight).

Dental film is supplied in packets (Figure 12-1) with an exterior nonabsorbent plastic envelope that acts as a barrier to moisture and light. Inside the plastic envelope, the film is enfolded in a black-paper light barrier. A thin sheet of lead foil is positioned behind the film to protect it from backscatter radiation from the patient's tissues, which can "fog" the film. This lead sheet is not thick enough to protect the patient from pass-through radiation. The lead sheets frequently have a stippled embossment pattern. If the film is inadvertently placed backward exposing the film through the lead, the stipple pattern and underexposed image on the developed radiograph alert the operator to the error.

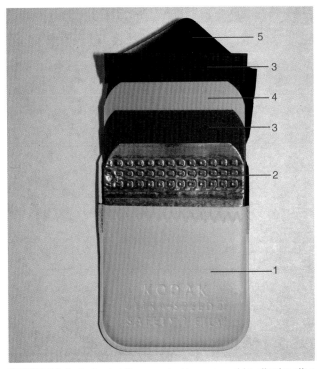

FIGURE 12-1 A dental film packet is opened to display the contents. *1,* Outer plastic wrap (back). *2,* Lead sheet. *3,* Black paper around the film. *4,* X-ray film. *5,* Lifted flap of plastic wrap.

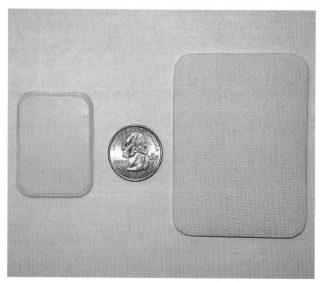

FIGURE 12-2 A quarter is positioned between size 2 (peri-apical) film (*left*) and size 4 (occlusal) film (*right*).

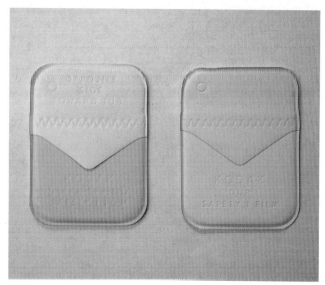

FIGURE 12-3 A film packet with normal x-ray–sensitive film (*left*) and a packet with visible light–sensitive duplicating film (*right*).

Dental film is available in sizes 0, 1, 2, 3, and 4. The most commonly used sizes in dogs and cats are the size 2 (periapical) film ($1\frac{1}{4} \times 1\frac{5}{8}$ inches, $31 \times 41$ mm) and the size 4 (occlusal) film ($2\frac{1}{4} \times 3$ inches, $57 \times 76$ mm) (Figure 12-2). Some operators find the size 0 ($\frac{7}{8} \times 1\frac{3}{8}$ inches) useful for cats and small dogs. Dental film is provided in single film packets, double film packets that make two identical radiographs, and duplicating film that is sensitive to incandescent light instead of x-rays. The backs of the packets are color coded to indicate the type of film inside (Figure 12-3).

The film is oriented in the patient's mouth with the front (Figure 12-4) toward the x-ray tube and the dimple (embossed circle in one corner) positioned coronally rather than apically. This is done to position the dimple away from the area of interest on the film.

Radiographs are best stored in film mounts where they can be correctly oriented and properly labeled. There are a number of mounts available for size 2 films (Figure 12-5). There are also larger cardboard mounts available for individual size 4 films. The mounted films can then be stored in marked envelopes and filed.

Standard size (nondental) x-ray film in a cassette with an intensifying screen is often used for radiography of the skull and temporomandibular joints (TMJs). Dental film, even the larger size 4 occlusal film, is usually too small to include both TMJs or the entire skull on one film.

## Positioning

Intraoral technique, using a dental x-ray machine with a mobile tube-head, is recommended for most dental and oral radiographs due to the ease of making excellent quality dental radiographs without superimposed anatomy. To use intraoral

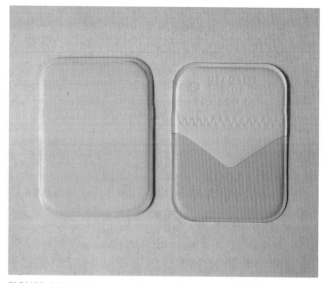

FIGURE 12-4 The front of the film packet (*left*) that is positioned toward the x-ray tube is relatively featureless except for the orientation dot. The back of the film packet (*right*) often has a tab to assist opening the packet and may also have other identifying marks.

technique, the dental film is placed inside the oral cavity instead of under the patient.

There are two basic positioning (film and tube-head) techniques used for making intraoral dental radiographs: parallel and bisecting angle. The parallel technique is used

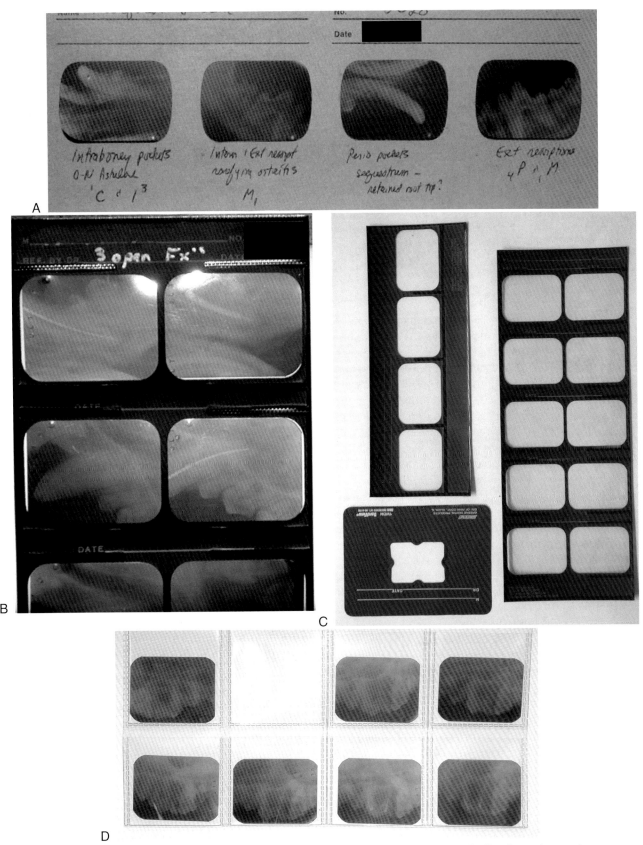

**FIGURE 12-5** Radiographs can be mounted for identification and storage. **A,** Cardboard mount. **B,**. Plastic mount. A white or silver marking pen can be used to write on the black plastic. **C,** Multiple configurations of plastic mounts. **D,** Clear plastic sheet with slots for holding radiographs. These can be cut to hold as many or as few radiographs as needed.

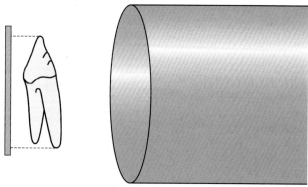

FIGURE 12-6 Parallel technique is the best positioning to avoid image distortion. The film is positioned parallel to the long axis of the tooth, and the x-ray beam is oriented perpendicular to both the tooth and the film.

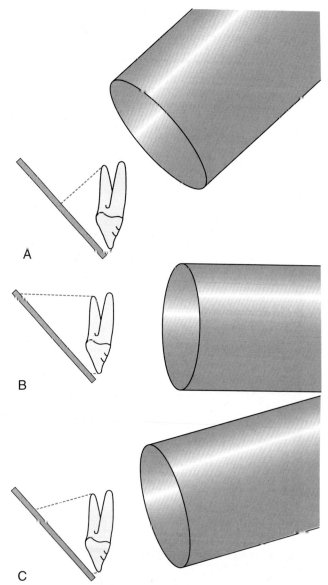

A

B

C

FIGURE 12-7 Bisecting angle technique is used when the film cannot be placed parallel to the long axis of the tooth due to anatomical interference. **A,** If the beam is oriented perpendicular to the film, it will make a foreshortened image on the film. **B,** If the beam is oriented perpendicular to the long axis of the tooth, it will make an elongated image on the film. **C,** If the beam is oriented half-way between these two (perpendicular to the line that bisects the angle between the axis of the tooth and the plane of the film), then the image will be the same length as the tooth.

whenever it is technically possible to place the film parallel to the axis of the tooth roots (Figure 12-6). In dogs and cats, this applies to the distal mandibular teeth, and sometimes the mandibular incisor and canine teeth depending on film placement and interference of the canine teeth and soft tissues. The film cannot be placed parallel to the teeth in the rostral mandibular premolar region due to the mandibular symphysis and angle of the roots relative to the oral surfaces. Similarly, film cannot be intraorally placed parallel to any of the maxillary teeth due to the position of the palate and lack of a high palatal vault in dogs and cats.

The bisecting angle technique uses a principle of geometry (the two sides of an isosceles triangle are equal in length) to prevent image elongation or foreshortening (Figure 12-7). The film is placed intraorally as close to the tooth as possible. Usually this involves placing the cusp tip at the extreme outside (aboral) edge of the film, or even off the film if it is not important to include the crown in the radiograph. This leaves the largest possible surface area of the film available for the roots. The film should not be bent, because any curvature of the film will cause distortion of the image. The x-ray beam (tube-head) is positioned perpendicular (at a right angle) to an imaginary line that bisects the angle formed between the film and the roots of the teeth being radiographed. Structures that are superimposed can be separated on the radiograph by shifting the tube-head in the third axis while maintaining the bisecting angle in the plane that includes the axis of the root and the edge (plane) of the film (Figure 12-8). For example, when making a radiograph of the premolar region, the tube-shift redirects the x-ray beam to a mesial-to-distal or distal-to-mesial direction while maintaining the bisecting angle position when viewed from the front of the patient (transverse plane). Shifting the tube mesially (mesiobuccal to distopalatal beam) moves objects that are closer to the tube-head distally on the radiograph image and objects that are closer to the film mesially. Conversely, when the tube-head is shifted distally (distobuccal to mesiopalatal beam), objects that are closer to the

tube-head will move mesially on the radiograph, while objects closer to the film will move distally on the radiograph. In other words, objects on the radiograph that move the same direction that the tube was shifted are on the palatal/lingual side, while objects that move the opposite direction from which the tube was shifted are on the buccal/labial side. A helpful acronym to remember this relationship is the "SLOB rule," which stands for **"Same Lingual Opposite Buccal"** (Figure 12-9).

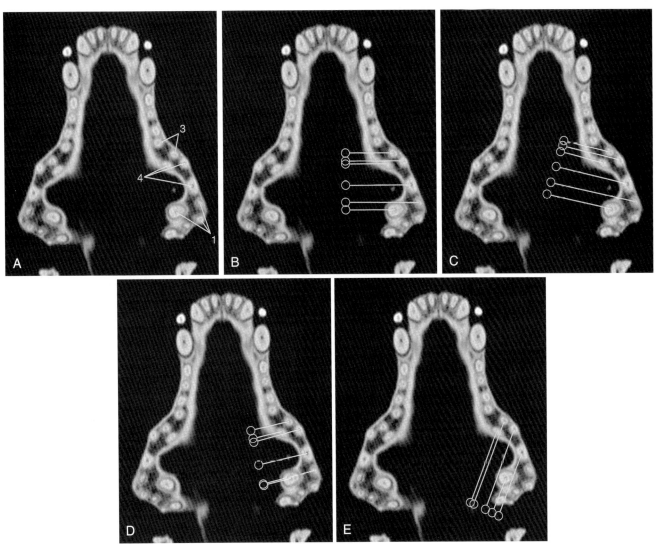

**FIGURE 12-8 Tube shift technique illustrated on a dorsal plane CT scan image. A,** The relationship of the roots of the maxillary fourth premolar tooth (4) to the roots of the third premolar (3) and first molar (1) varies between individuals depending on size, tooth crowding, and head shape. **B,** In the standard orientation of the x-ray beam perpendicular to the film in the dorsal plane and using bisecting angle in the transverse plane, the roots are projected onto the film as indicated by the circles. **C,** While maintaining the bisecting angle in the transverse plane, the tube-head is shifted caudally (distally) to separate the distal root of the fourth premolar from the roots of the first molar. **D,** While maintaining the bisecting angle in the transverse plane, the tube-head is shifted rostrally (mesially) to separate the mesiobuccal root of the fourth premolar from the palatal root of the same tooth. **E,** If the tube is shifted too far rostrally, and in some brachycephalic breeds, the palatal root may be superimposed over the distal root of the third premolar tooth.

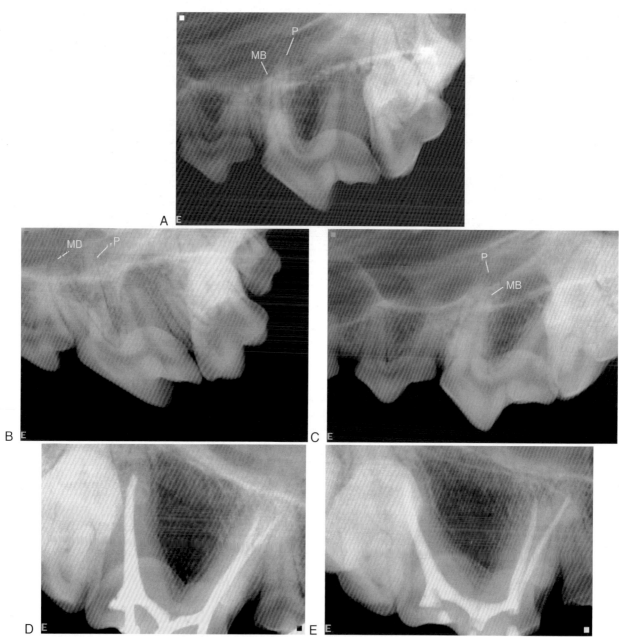

**FIGURE 12-9  A,** Normal laterally positioned radiograph of the maxillary fourth premolar tooth. There is superimposition of the mesiobuccal (MB) and palatal (P) roots. **B,** The tube was shifted caudally (distally), moving the palatal root distally on the image. **C,** The tube was shifted rostrally (mesially), moving the palatal root mesially on the image. **D,** Anatomy varies between individuals. In this patient, the distal root is clearly seen; part of the MB and P roots are superimposed, and they diverge apically. **E,** Moving the tube-head rostrally (mesially) separates the MB from the P root, but now the distal root is superimposed over the first molar. Two views are sometimes required to visualize all roots. **D** was a procedural film and **E** was the postoperative film.

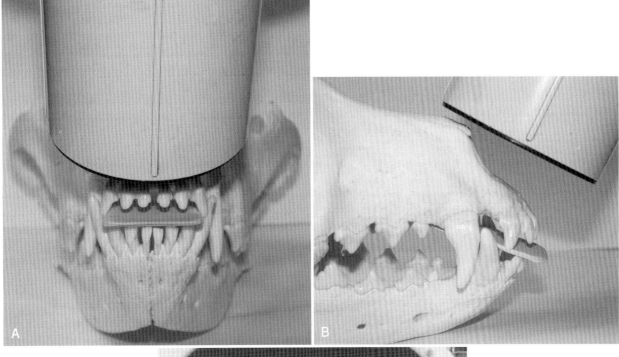

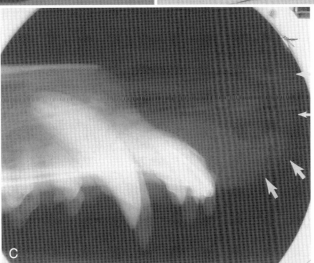

FIGURE 12-10 Maxillary incisors. **A,** On a small-to-medium sized dog, the x-ray beam should be perpendicular to the film and parallel to the line that connects the maxillary midline to the mandibular midline when viewed from the front. **B,** Viewed from the side, the x-ray beam is perpendicular to an imaginary line that bisects the angle made by the film and the tooth root axis. **C,** The axis of the roots, not the crowns, is used when determining the bisecting angle. On this radiograph, the soft tissue of the nose is visible, (*arrows*), with a very different profile from the bone and incisor roots.

## POSITIONING FOR MAKING RADIOGRAPHS OF THE DOG

In discussing patient positioning, the "angle" will be understood to mean the angle made between the line of the longitudinal axis of the tooth root and the plane of the film. A very handy film-positioning device is a wadded paper towel or part of a paper towel (the paper towel film positioning device [PTFPD]). It is soft enough to prevent bending of the film, adaptable to all sizes of patients, inexpensive, readily available, and disposable.

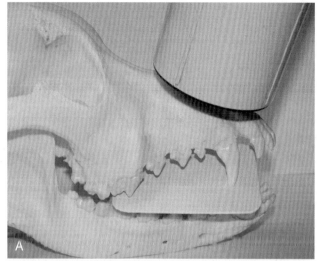

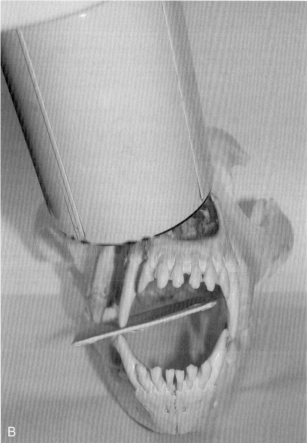

FIGURE 12-11 **Maxillary canine. A,** Viewed from the side, the x-ray beam is perpendicular to an imaginary line that bisects the angle made by the film and the tooth root axis. The tooth root can usually be located by palpating the prominent canine root eminence (in the veterinary literature, this is sometimes called the *jugum,* a term that refers to the trough between eminences in human anatomy). **B,** Viewed from the front, the x-ray beam is slightly lateral from dorsoventral projection.

## Maxillary Incisor Teeth (Figure 12-10)

One radiograph can include all the maxillary incisor teeth of small-to-medium breeds. The film is placed with the incisor cusp tips along the short side of the film that has the dimple. The tube is positioned perpendicular to the film when viewed from the front and to bisect the angle when viewed from the side. Large-breed dogs may require a separate radiograph for the third incisor teeth, with the tube-head angled from slightly more lateral when viewed from the front.

## Maxillary Canine Teeth (Figure 12-11)

Size 4 (occlusal) film is helpful to avoid missing the root apex. The film is placed horizontally in the mouth with the canine cusp tip on the outside (aboral) rostral corner of the film. The tube is positioned to bisect the angle when viewed from the side, and angled laterally from a dorsoventral (DV) position when viewed from the front. This projects the root tip to the opposite corner of the film from the cusp tip.

## Maxillary Premolars (Figure 12-12)

The first through third premolars are often included on one image, and a separate radiograph is made of the fourth premolar. On small dogs, it may be possible to include all the premolars on a single radiograph. The tube is positioned to bisect the angle when viewed from the front and perpendicular to the film and alveolar ridge when viewed from the top or side. Tube-shift can be performed as described above to separate superimposed structures on the image.

## Maxillary Molar Teeth (Figure 12-13)

The alveolar arch curves medially behind the premolars in most dogs (see Figure 12-8). The tube is positioned to bisect the angle when viewed from rostrolateral (from the mesial contact surface of the tooth), and perpendicular to the film, the buccal surface of the molars and alveolar ridge when viewed from the top.

## Mandibular Incisor Teeth (Figure 12-14)

One radiograph can include all the incisor teeth. The film is placed with the incisor cusp tips along the short side of the film. The tube is positioned perpendicular to the film when viewed from the front and to bisect the angle when viewed from the side.

## Mandibular Canine Teeth (Figure 12-15)

One radiograph can include the apices of both canine teeth. The positioning is similar to that for the mandibular incisors but angled slightly more ventrodorsally. The tube is positioned to bisect the angle when viewed from the side. For dedicated radiographs of one canine tooth (for example, during endodontic treatment) and to prevent superimposition of the first premolar tooth, the tube can be angled from slightly lateral rather than perpendicular when viewed from the front.

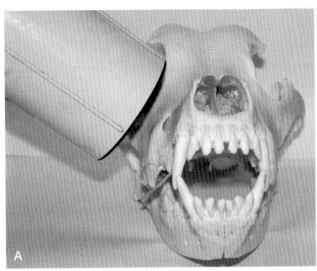

FIGURE 12-12 **Maxillary premolars. A,** Viewed from the front, the x-ray beam is perpendicular to an imaginary line that bisects the angle made by the film and the axes of the tooth roots. **B,** Viewed from the top, the x-ray beam is perpendicular to the plane of the film and the plane of the tooth roots and alveolar ridge. **C,** Shifting the tube caudally (distally) separates the distal root of the fourth premolar from the first molar and moves the palatal root distally on the radiograph. **D,** Shifting the tube rostrally (mesially) separates the mesiobuccal and palatal roots of the fourth premolar and moves the palatal root mesially on the radiograph.

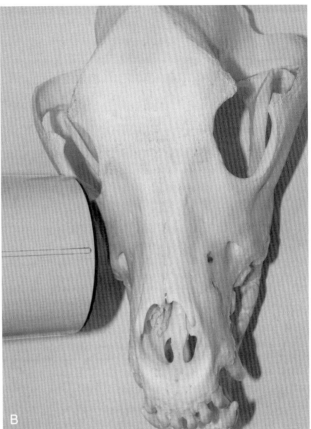

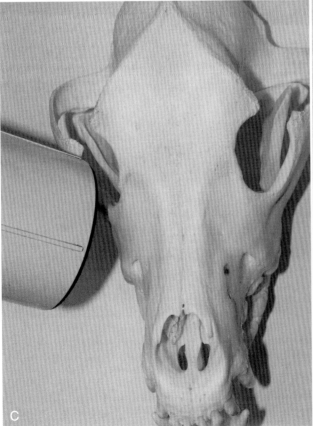

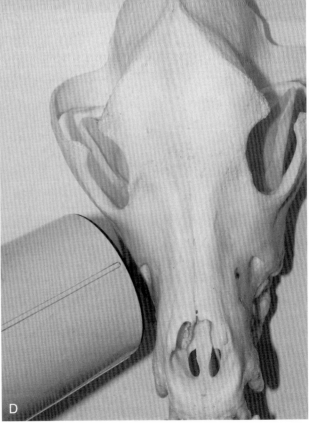

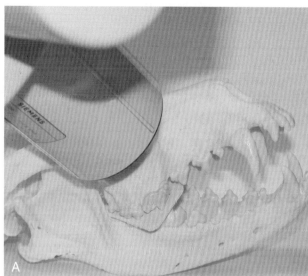

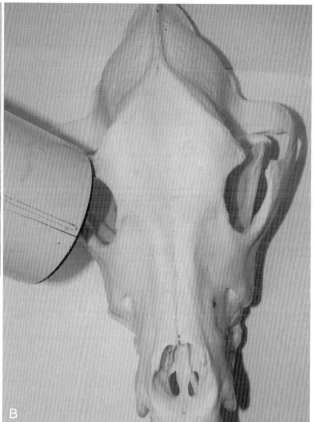

FIGURE 12-13 Maxillary molars. A, Viewed from the side, the x-ray beam is perpendicular to an imaginary line that bisects the angle made by the plane of the film and the axes of the tooth roots. B, Viewed from the top, the x-ray beam is perpendicular to the plane of the film, the plane of the tooth roots and alveolar ridge. The angle is from the caudalateral.

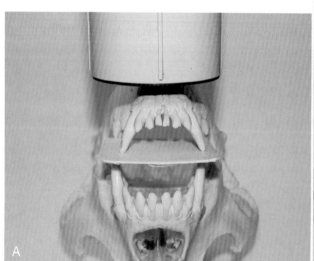

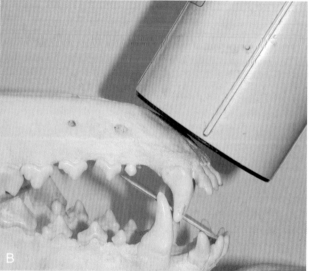

FIGURE 12-14 Mandibular incisors. A, The x-ray beam is perpendicular to the film and parallel to the line that connects the maxillary midline to the mandibular midline when viewed from the front. B, Viewed from the side, the x-ray beam is perpendicular to an imaginary line that bisects the angle made by the film and the tooth root axis. With the angle of the roots in this case, it is nearly parallel technique.

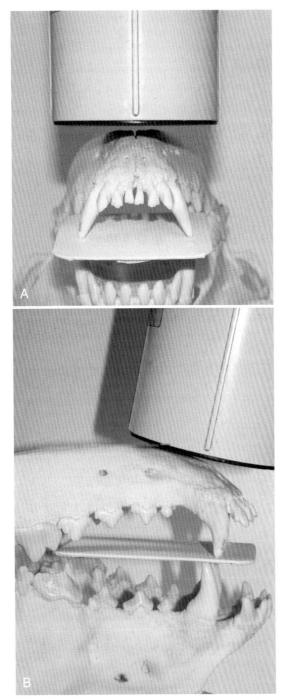

FIGURE 12-15 **Mandibular canines. A,** The x-ray beam is perpendicular to the film and parallel to the line that connects the maxillary midline to the mandibular midline when viewed from the front. **B,** Viewed from the side, the x-ray beam is perpendicular to an imaginary line that bisects the angle made by the film and the axis of the roots (not the crowns) of the canine teeth.

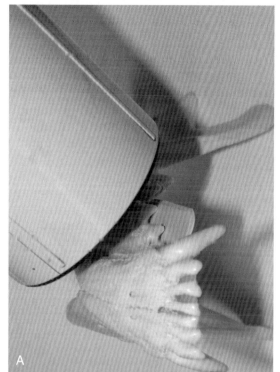

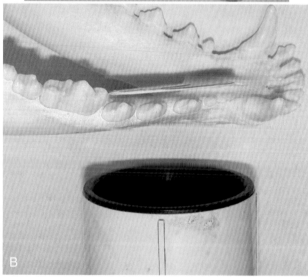

FIGURE 12-16 Rostral (mesial) mandibular premolars. **A,** Viewed from the front, the x-ray beam is perpendicular to an imaginary line that bisects the angle made by the film and the axes of the tooth roots. The tube may need to be shifted to a more ventral position to project the root of the first premolar coronally (dorsally) onto the x-ray film. **B,** Viewed from the side, the x-ray beam is perpendicular to the plane of the film and the plane of the tooth roots.

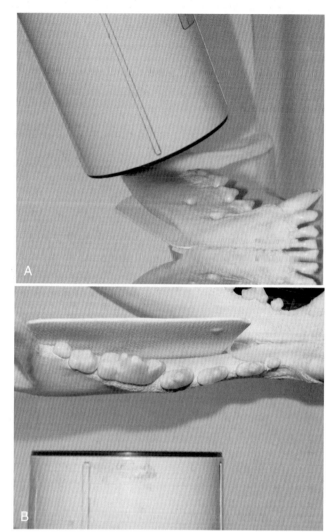

FIGURE 12-17 Caudal (distal) mandibular premolar and molar teeth. Parallel technique is used, positioning the x-ray beam perpendicular to the plane of the film and the plane of the tooth roots when viewed from all angles. **A,** When viewed from the front this gives the appearance of a ventrolateral-to-dorsolingual angle because the roots and the film converge ventrally (apically). **B,** Dorsal (occlusal) view.

### Rostral (Mesial) Mandibular Premolar Teeth (First and Second) (Figure 12-16)

The rostral premolar teeth are adjacent to the symphysis, requiring the film to be placed along the floor of the mouth. The tube is positioned to bisect the angle when viewed from the front, and perpendicular to the film when viewed from the side or top.

### Caudal (Distal) Mandibular Premolar and Molar Teeth (Figure 12-17)

This is the one region in which parallel technique can routinely be used. The film is placed into the space between the tongue and the lingual surface of the mandible, posi-

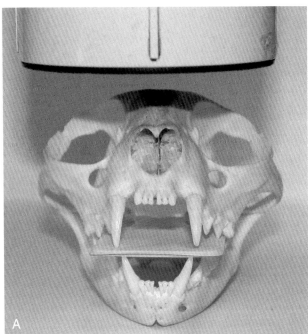

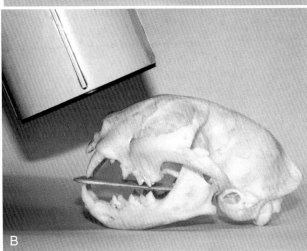

**FIGURE 12-18** Cat: maxillary incisors. **A,** The x-ray beam is perpendicular to the film and parallel to the line that would connect the maxillary midline to the mandibular midline when viewed from the front. **B,** Viewed from the side, the x-ray beam is perpendicular to an imaginary line that bisects the angle made by the film and the axes of the tooth roots.

tioned apically so the cusp tip is level with the top of the film. The edge of the film can be felt between the mandibles to assure it is placed sufficiently apically to include the roots and surrounding bone. The tube is positioned perpendicular to the plane of the tooth roots and to the film.

## POSITIONING FOR MAKING RADIOGRAPHS OF THE CAT

Size 2 films are used for all intraoral radiographs of the cat except for radiographs of the nasal cavity. The tube and film position for making radiographs of the maxillary incisor and canine teeth are positioned the same as for dogs

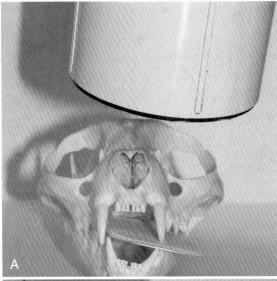

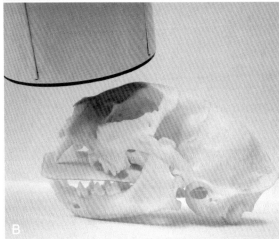

**FIGURE 12-19** Cat: maxillary canine. **A,** Viewed from the front, the x-ray beam is slightly lateral from dorsoventral projection. **B,** Viewed from the side, the x-ray beam is perpendicular to an imaginary line that bisects the angle made by the film and the tooth root axis.

(Figures 12-18 and 12-19). Positioning for the maxillary premolar teeth is similar to that for the dog (Figure 12-20) but is modified by lowering the tube-head ventrally to drop the x-ray beam under the zygomatic arch (Figure 12-21). This will result in slight, but acceptable, elongation of the roots. The mandibular incisor teeth and canine teeth can be included in a single radiograph that is positioned similar to that for dogs (Figure 12-22). Positioning for the mandibular premolars and molar is also similar to that for dogs (Figure 12-23).

## EXTRAORAL TECHNIQUE

If a dedicated dental x-ray machine is not available, extraoral radiographs of dental structures can be made using either dental film or standard full-sized x-ray film in

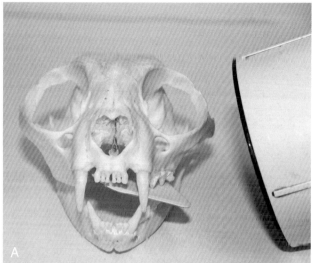

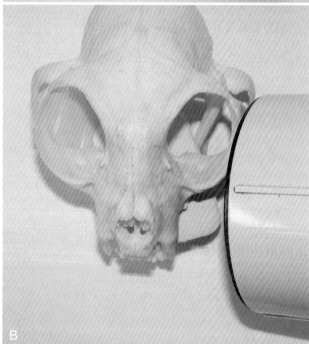

**FIGURE 12-20**  Cat: maxillary premolars and molar. **A,** Viewed from the front, the x-ray beam is not directly perpendicular to the imaginary line that bisects the angle made by the film and the axes of the tooth roots. The tube is shifted ventral (more lateral projection than bisecting angle) to avoid superimposition of the zygomatic arch. **B,** Viewed from the top, the x-ray beam is perpendicular to the plane of the film and the plane of the tooth roots and alveolar ridge. The film is skewed to fit maximally in the oral cavity. The long side of the film is placed against the palatal surfaces of the premolars of the contralateral quadrant, and the short side is placed against the distal surface of the ipsilateral canine tooth.

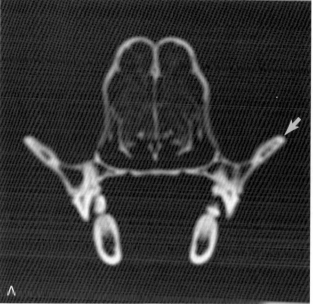

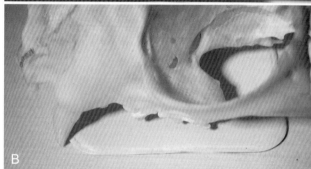

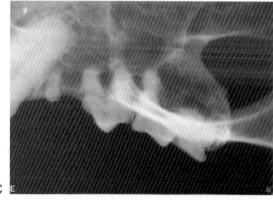

**FIGURE 12-21**  Cat: superimposition of the zygomatic arch. **A,** Transverse plane CT scan image of a cat skull at the level of the mesial and palatal roots of the maxillary fourth premolar tooth. The primary beam (*arrow*) at an angle for normal bisecting angle technique travels through the zygomatic arch. **B,** View of the skull perpendicular to the bisecting angle. **C,** On a radiograph using the bisecting angle technique some roots are superimposed over the zygomatic arch.

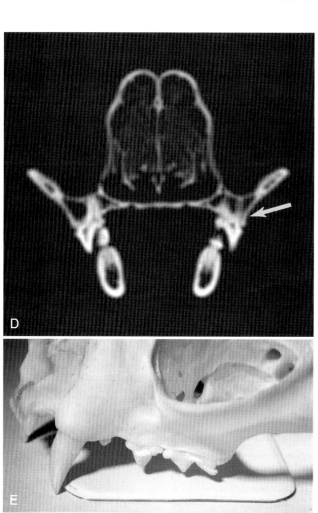

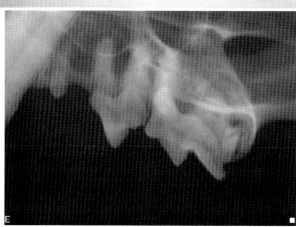

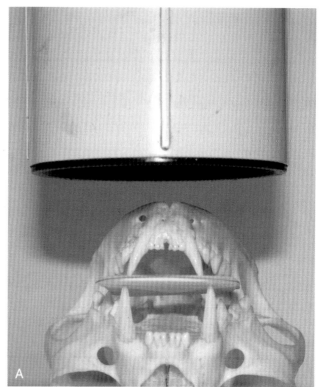

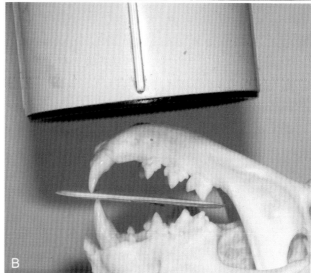

**FIGURE 12-21, cont'd  D,** Transverse plane CT scan image of a cat skull at the level of the mesial and palatal roots of the maxillary fourth premolar tooth. The primary beam (*arrow*) with the tube shifted ventrally from the angle for bisecting angle technique travels under the zygomatic arch. **E,** View of the skull from the more horizontal angle in **D. F,** On a radiograph using the more horizontal angle, the zygomatic arch is shifted dorsally (apically) and the less tangential angle decreases its radiopacity.

**FIGURE 12-22  Cat: mandibular incisors and canines. A,** The x-ray beam is perpendicular to the film and parallel to the line that would connect the maxillary midline to the mandibular midline when viewed from the front. **B,** Viewed from the side, the x-ray beam is perpendicular to an imaginary line that bisects the angle made by the film and the axes of the tooth roots.

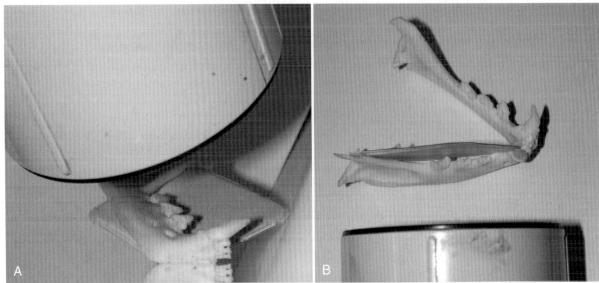

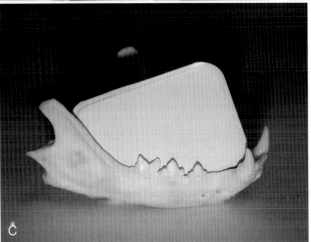

**FIGURE 12-23 Cat: mandibular premolars and molar.** Parallel technique is used, positioning the x-ray beam perpendicular to the plane of the film and the plane of the tooth roots when viewed from all angles. **A,** When viewed from the front this gives the appearance of a ventrolateral-to-dorsolingual angle since the roots and the film converge ventrally (apically). **B,** Viewed from the side. **C,** The film is placed as far back in the mouth as possible with the caudal part of the ventral edge extending ventrally to the ventral cortex, and the rostral part limited by the symphysis. Clinically, this is accomplished by placing the long edge of the film under the tie material used to secure the endotracheal tube in position.

cassettes. The detail on radiographs made using extraoral technique is generally not as good as those made using intraoral technique. Positioning is more difficult when using a stationary tube-head to make extraoral dental radiographs. The mouth is opened wide and the head is positioned obliquely to prevent superimposition of the contralateral maxillary or mandibular dentition (Figure 12-24).

## POSITIONING FOR MAKING TEMPOROMANDIBULAR JOINT RADIOGRAPHS USING DENTAL FILM

Radiographic views of the TMJ are taken with the x-ray beam directed in a DV or lateral direction through the TMJ. The TMJs may both be projected on a single large film or

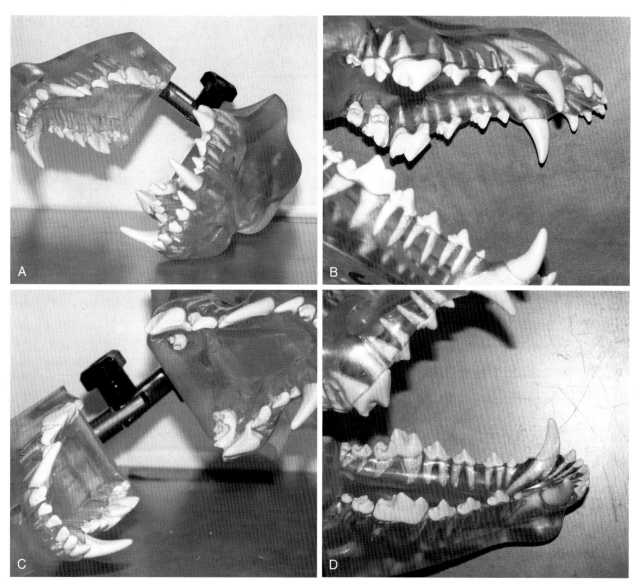

**FIGURE 12-24 Extraoral technique demonstrated with clear dog models on an x-ray cassette. A,** To radiograph the maxillary premolar and molar teeth, the quadrant to be radiographed is placed down on the cassette. The head is positioned oblique enough to rotate the contralateral maxillary quadrant (1) dorsally, and the mouth is opened wide enough to move the contralateral mandible (2) ventrally, to prevent superimposition. **B,** The view of the maxillary quadrant from the perspective of the x-ray tube. **C,** To radiograph the mandibular premolar and molar teeth, the head is positioned oblique enough to rotate the contralateral mandible (2) ventrally, and the mouth is opened wide enough to move the contralateral maxillary quadrant (1) dorsally, to prevent superimposition. **D,** View of the mandibular quadrant from the perspective of the x-ray tube.

individually projected on a smaller dental film or sensor. The film is placed extraorally when making TMJ radiographs.

The DV view is made with the patient positioned in sternal recumbency with the head and neck extended. The head should be stabilized in a position that would place both TMJs equal distance from the plane of the radiograph film and the palate/mandible parallel to the radiographic film. The x-ray beam is perpendicular to the x-ray film (Figure 12-25). The DV radiograph of the TMJ is helpful in diagnosing fractures, luxations, and subluxations of the TMJ.

To make a lateral view of the TMJ, the patient is first placed in lateral recumbency with the head positioned so the midline of the maxilla is parallel with the x-ray film. In this position, the TMJs are directly superimposed over each

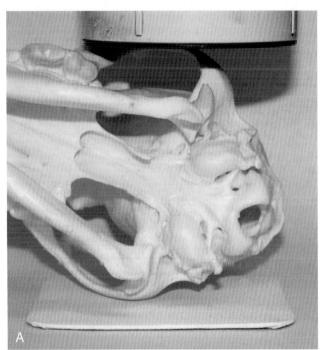

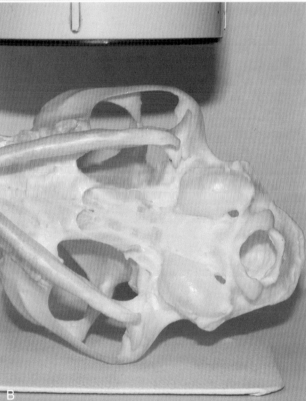

FIGURE 12-26 Positioning for a lateral view of the TMJ is the same for dogs and cats. **A,** Ventral view of the positioning in a dog illustrating the orientation of the film, head, TMJs, and tube-head. **B,** Positioning illustrated in a cat.

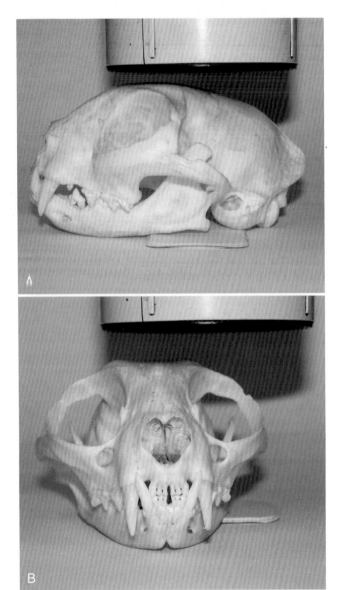

FIGURE 12-25 Positioning for a dorsoventral view of the TMJ is the same for cats and dogs. **A,** Lateral view of the positioning of the film, head, and tube-head. **B,** Front view of the positioning of the film, head, and tube-head.

other. Then the nose is elevated approximately 30 degrees to separate the TMJs (Figure 12-26). In lateral recumbency, elevating the nose moves the TMJ closest to the film forward of the TMJ farthest from the film.

A slightly different view (intraorbital view) of the TMJ can be made with the x-ray beam directed anterior to posterior through the orbit. The patient is positioned as for a DV view. The tube-head is positioned at a 45-degree angle to the x-ray film viewed from the side and angled 10 to 15 degrees toward the midline (Figure 12-27).

## Exposure Times

The exposure times required for dental radiographs vary depending on the tissue thickness, cone length (focal-film distance), and film sensitivity. Generally, for most modern dental x-ray machines, an exposure time between 0.08 second and 0.6 second for D-speed through F-speed films is needed. In most equipment configurations, only six settings are required for all needs—an upper and lower exposure time each for cats, for small dogs, and for large dogs.

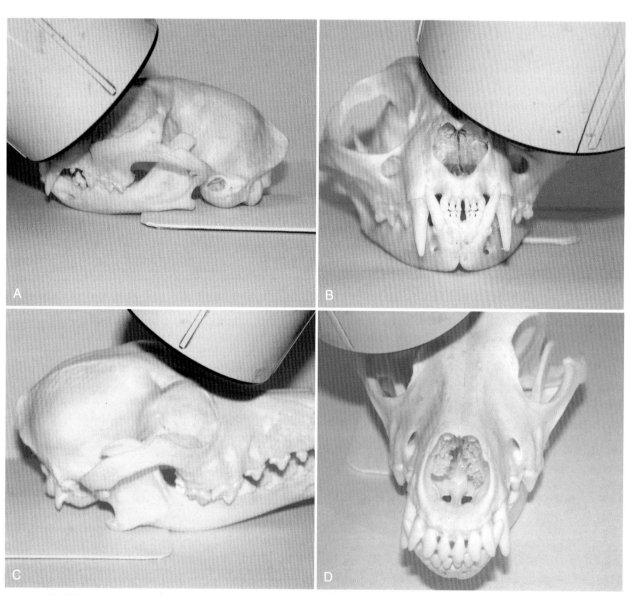

**FIGURE 12-27 Intraorbital view of the TMJ in dogs and cats. A,** Lateral view to illustrate the positioning of the tube-head and x-ray film in a cat. **B,** Front view of the positioning of the tube-head angled slightly (10 to 15 degrees) toward the midline in a cat. **C,** Lateral view to illustrate the positioning of the tube-head and x-ray film in a dog. **D,** Front view of the positioning of the tube-head angled slightly (10 to 15 degrees) toward the midline in a dog.

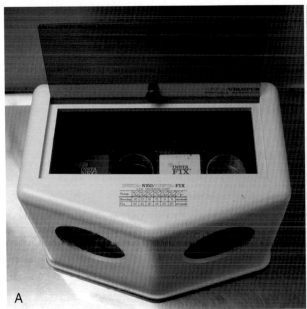

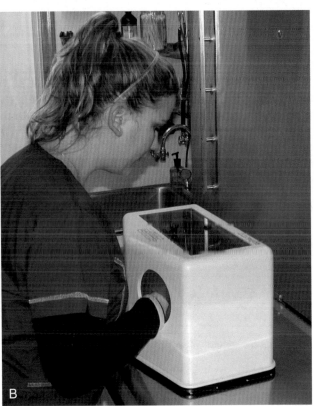

**FIGURE 12-28** **Chair side developer. A,** The lid is open to show the containers with chemicals. The developer and fixer containers have tight-fitting lids. **B,** The operator's hands enter through the lightproof portals to develop the films. A light-filtering lid allows visualization during use.

Most digital radiography equipment uses a sensor and software that require a tenth of the radiation needed to expose D-speed film, generally requiring exposure times between 0.02 and 0.06 second. However, this is not universal and some manufacturers make digital equipment that requires higher levels of radiation than this.

## Processing

Errors made during film processing can greatly contribute to inaccurate interpretation. Dental films can be developed using a chair-side developing system (Figure 12-28), regular dip-tanks, small containers in the darkroom containing dental rapid developers and fixers, or an automatic processor.

Automatic processors specifically designed for dental films are expensive and may not be practical for the veterinarian. The automatic processor designed to develop regular x-ray film can also be used to develop dental radiographs by taping the dental film to a leader film that pulls it through the automatic processor. The area under the tape does not develop the latent image, and there is a risk of the dental film detaching from the leader film and becoming lost in the processor, necessitating removal to prevent it from adhering to, and ruining, a subsequent film.

Chair-side developers are the most practical for most practices, allowing fast developing without leaving the dental operatory. There are a few available. Those that have containers that are large enough to accept size 4 film are recommended. Depending on the solution and temperature, the film is swirled in the rapid developer for 10 to 40 seconds. It is then rinsed in water and placed in the fixer for twice as long as it was in the developer. After rinsing and reading, it is generally recommended to place the radiograph in fresh water for 10 minutes to ensure that there are no residual chemicals on the emulsion surface prior to drying.

## Exposure Errors (Table 12-1)

| TABLE 12-1 Exposure Errors | | |
|---|---|---|
| **PROBLEM** | **CAUSE** | **RESOLUTION** |
| Dark film | Overexposed | Decease exposure time |
| Light film | Underexposed | Increase exposure time |

## Processing Errors (Table 12-2; Figure 12-29)

**TABLE 12-2** Processing Errors

| PROBLEM | CAUSE | RESOLUTION |
|---|---|---|
| Black spots | Developer contamination prior to processing | Careful processing |
| Brown discoloration | Incomplete fixing or rinsing | Check fluid temperature, expiration, and timing |
| Clear area along one edge | Processing fluid level low | Add fluids to containers |
| Dark film (not overexposed) | Overdeveloped | Decrease processing times |
| Entire film clear | Emulsion detached from film or unexposed film | Do not soak in water too long |
| Fingerprints | Improper film handling with contaminated fingers | Use film hanger to transfer film |
| Fogged film | Light contamination or overprocessing | Check correct light filter on chair side developer, processing times, fluid temp |
| Frosted film surface | Incomplete rinsing | Verify fluids are not depleted and rinsing is adequate |
| Green discolored areas | Films in contact during processing | Keep films separated from each other during processing |
| Incomplete variable processing | Paper processed with the film | Carefully process only film |
| Light film (not underexposed) | Underprocessed | Warm or replace fluids |
| Mottled areas of underexposure and overexposure | Poorly mixed fluids with temperature variances | Agitate fluids prior to processing |
| Small white circles | Bubbles in processing solution | Do not use rough agitation |
| Streaks | Inadequate processing or fluid contamination | Change fluids or examine processing time |
| Thick white lines | Scratched emulsion during processing | Careful processing |
| White spots | Fixer contamination prior to processing | Careful processing |

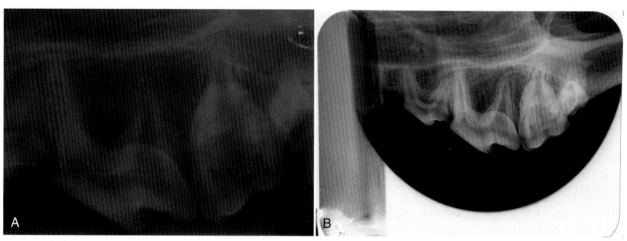

FIGURE 12-29 Processing errors. **A,** Incomplete fixing. **B,** The lines on the left were caused by low fluid levels.

*Continued.*

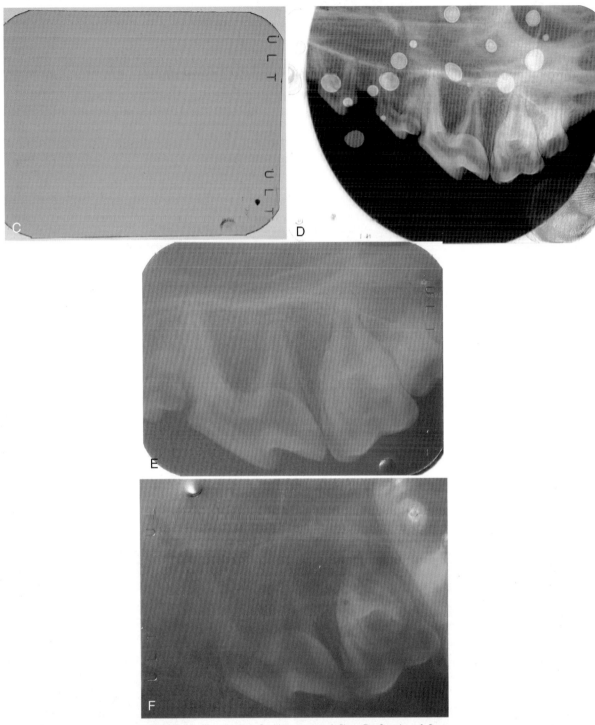

**FIGURE 12-29, cont'd C,** Unexposed film. **D,** Spots of fixer contaminated the film prior to processing. There is also a fingerprint from a finger that had fixer on the surface. **E,** Poor rinse. **F,** Processed without removing the black light-barrier paper.

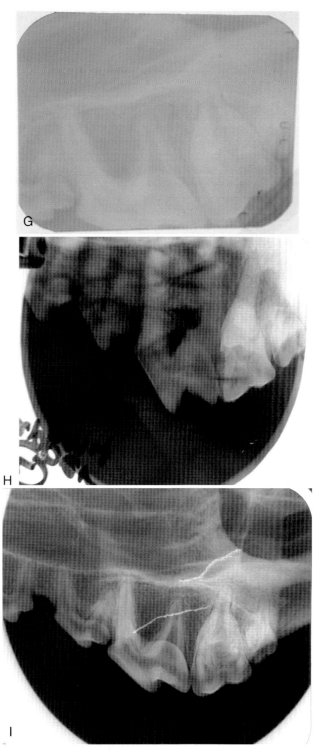

**FIGURE 12-29, cont'd G,** Poorly developed. **H,** Poorly mixed fluids with varying temperature. **I,** Scratched emulsion during processing.

## Positioning Errors (Table 12-3; Figure 12-30)

### TABLE 12-3 Positioning Errors

| PROBLEM | CAUSE | RESOLUTION |
|---|---|---|
| Area of interest not on image | Positioning error | Change tube angle or film position or both |
| Black circle in corner over image | Film dimple not placed coronally | Position film with dimple toward the crowns |
| Blurred image | Motion of patient or tube-head | Anesthesia, adjust suspension arm |
| Clear circular perimeter | Cone cut | Position tube over entire film |
| Dark crescents or lines | Sharp bend or pressure on film after exposing but before processing | Handle film carefully prior to processing |
| Elongated image | Tube angle too shallow (too perpendicular to tooth when bisecting angle) | Increase angle to more vertical position |
| Foreshortened image | Tube angle too steep (too perpendicular to film when bisecting angle) | Drop angle to more lateral position |
| Image distortion | Bent film, positioning error | Repeat with correct positioning and non-bent film |
| Opacities | Undesired materials included in x-ray field | Remove foreign materials from between the x-ray tube and the film |
| Roots angled from crowns | Tube angulation problem | Shift tube to the direction of root angulation |
| Stipple pattern on light film | Film placed backward | Repeat with correct placement |
| Superimposed structures | Summation effect | Additional exposures with tube shifted mesial or distal |
| White crescents or lines | Sharp bend or pressure on film prior to exposing | Handle film carefully prior to exposure |

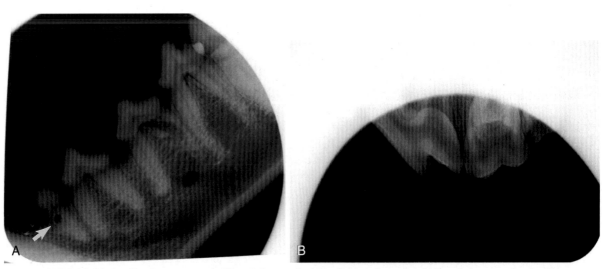

**FIGURE 12-30 Positioning errors. A,** Film dot superimposed over the root of the first premolar tooth. **B,** Cone cut.

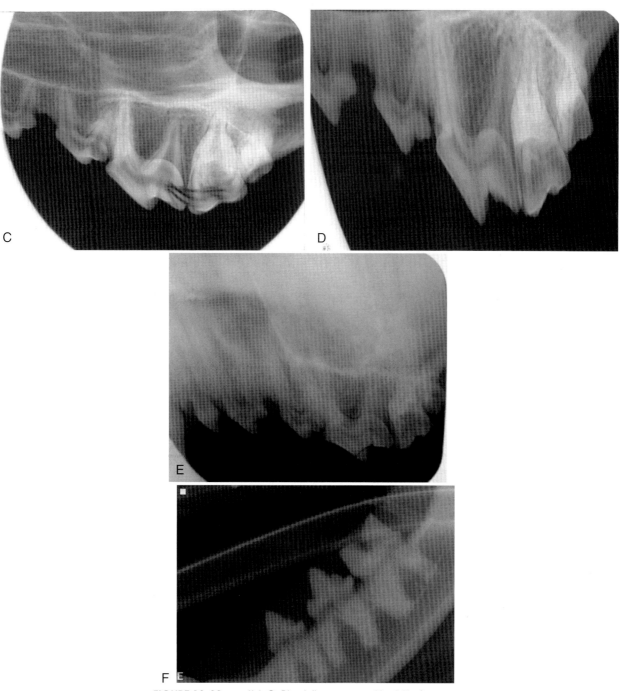

**FIGURE 12-30, cont'd  C,** Black lines caused by bite force on film. **D,** Image elongation caused by a tube angle too perpendicular to the tooth axis and too parallel to the film. **E,** Bent film made the tooth crowns appear normal but the roots are very long and distorted. **F,** Linear opacity is the endotracheal tube positioned between the x-ray tube and the sensor.

*Continued.*

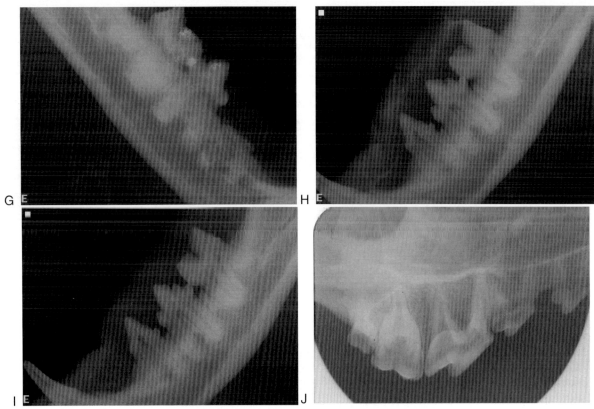

**FIGURE 12-30, cont'd G,** White spots are radiopaque prophy paste. **H,** Radiopacity coronal to the teeth is caused by water-soaked long hair. **I,** This radiograph of the patient from **H** made after the hair was dried. **J,** The film was placed backward, making an underexposed image with a stipple pattern.

## SUGGESTED READINGS

Mulligan TW, Aller MS, Williams CA: *Atlas of canine and feline dental radiography,* Trenton, NJ, 1998, Veterinary Learning Systems.

Oakes A: Introduction. In: DeForge DH, Colmery BH, editors: *An atlas of veterinary dental radiology,* Ames, IA, 2000, Iowa State University Press.

Whaites E: *Essentials of dental radiography and radiology,* ed 3, New York, 2002, Churchill Livingstone.

Wiggs RB, Lobprise HB: *Veterinary dentistry principles and practice,* Philadelphia, 1997, Lippincott–Raven.

CHAPTER 13

# Equipment

Radiographs are images of the shadows made when x-rays (electromagnetic waves of pure energy that generate both electrical and magnetic fields) incompletely and differentially penetrate imaged objects. X-rays that are able to pass through the object interact with the film or sensor, while those that are absorbed or deflected by radiodense objects do not. This creates a shadow image on the film or sensor that consists of a "gray scale" of black through white that corresponds to x-rays traveling through the object uninterrupted (black) through complete blocking (white) and shades of gray between. This scale can have many different levels of gray (long scale) with very subtle differences between them, or it can have very few gradations of gray (short scale) that are much more distinct.

Dental x-ray machines generate the x-rays using very compact equipment that includes a generator, a tube head, and a control panel.

## Dental Radiograph Machines

X-ray equipment for general radiography in most veterinary facilities consists of a stationary tube head suspended over a patient-positioning table. Dental radiographs can be made using this equipment using extraoral technique (see Chapter 12). However, a dedicated dental x-ray machine greatly facilitates creating dental and oral radiographs. Intraoral technique with a dedicated dental x-ray machine provides high-quality images without leaving the dental operatory. The purchase cost is a modest investment with a fast return when used as it should be.

### GENERATOR

The generator sends a precise quantity and quality of energy to the tube head, stimulating the firing of electrons toward a target (anode) in the tube head. The quantity of electrons is determined by the amperage and exposure time (milliampere-seconds, or mAs), and their acceleration

energy toward the target is determined by the applied voltage (kVp). The target takes the delivered quantity of electrons and converts their energy into x-ray photons. Some dental x-ray units may have set kVp and milliamperage (mA) values, while others allow the operator to select an mA setting between 7 and 15 mA and a kVp setting between 60 and 90 kVp. Higher kVp and lower mAs make fewer x-rays with higher penetrating ability. In contrast to this, using a low kVp and a high mAs tends to produce images using more x-rays but with less penetrating ability. A balance needs to be struck between images that are pleasing to view with high contrast and very black-and-white character, and images that are more challenging to interpret due to the additional shadows and more shades of gray but also contain more diagnostic information (Figure 13-1). All units allow the operator to select an exposure time, either directly or indirectly. The exposure time may be in fractions of a second, or it may be in "pulses" that are 1/60th of a second.

### CONTROL UNIT AND INTERFACE

The user interfaces vary between units. The simplest units with a set kVp and mA have only a power button, a digital timer exposure control, and an exposure button (Figure 13-2, A). Others do not allow direct selection of exposure time, instead using an anatomical interface that requires the operator to select the size and species of the patient and the specific tooth being radiographed (Figure 13-2, B). Many now allow either anatomical selection or direct timer selection (Figure 13-2, C–F). Those with the anatomic interface also have some way of setting the equipment to the operator's specific site variables (cone length, film speed, or sensor type) that affect the amount of radiation needed for diagnostic images. The exposure button on the control unit needs to be pressed throughout the exposure. Removing pressure mid-exposure interrupts the generation of x-rays and usually generates a machine error code to warn the operator of the underexposure. This is designed as a safety precaution.

255

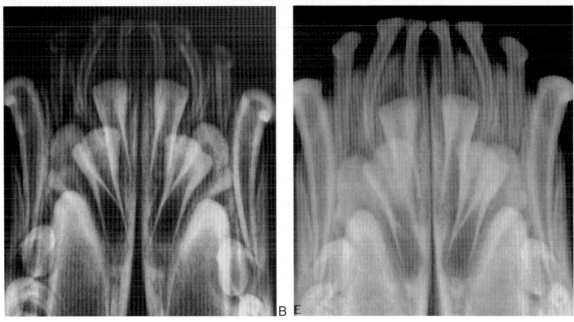

FIGURE 13-1 **High-contrast versus low-contrast image. A,** At first glance, this image is pleasing to view due to the clarity and ease of identifying bony structures. **B,** A lower contrast image is less clear but contains far more information. Septal bone can now be seen between the deciduous incisor teeth.

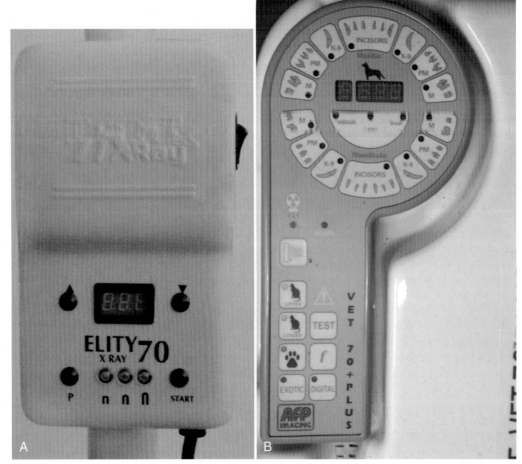

FIGURE 13-2 **Control units. A,** A simple control allowing the user to set the exposure time and make the radiograph. **B,** An anatomical interface without timer selector.

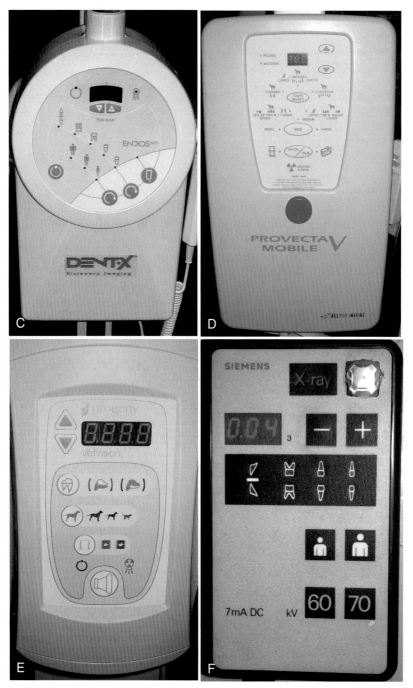

**FIGURE 13-2, cont'd C–E,** Anatomical interface with timer selector. **F,** The authors' unit, which has been in service for more than 12 years, has a timer and kV selector. The only buttons used are the exposure time selector and the activation button. The plastic covering has long ago worn off the exposure button.

## TUBE HEAD

The tube head of a dental x-ray unit is attached by a universal mount to a long jointed arm (Figure 13-3). The head contains the x-ray tube and associated electronics. The x-ray beam exits through a position-indicating device (PID), often called the "cone." The term "cone" was used because earlier models had a cone-shaped PID with the apex pointing toward the object to be radiographed. Modern PIDs are hollow cylinders of varying lengths. The PID length determines the focal-film distance (FFD [the distance from the focal spot on the target to the film or sensor]) because it is placed as close as possible to the patient when making a radiograph. Although a short cone technically allows more beam divergence and scatter exposure of the patient than a long-cone technique, it

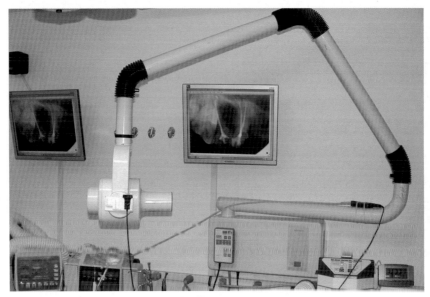

FIGURE 13-3 Wall-mounted dental x-ray unit with the head supported on a jointed positioning arm.

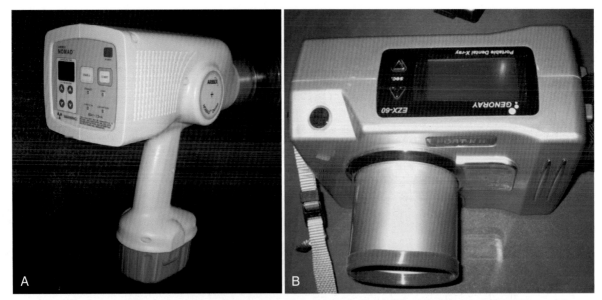

FIGURE 13-4 Hand-held portable x-ray machines the size of a portable drill (**A**) or camera (**B**) could prove valuable for a mobile practice.

provides the advantage of using less radiation by a factor of the square of the decreased distance. In other words, a long-cone technique at 16-inch FFD requires four times more radiation than a short-cone technique at an 8-inch FFD.

## MOUNTING

Dental x-ray machines can be wall or ceiling mounted (see Figure 13-3), stand supported, or hand-held (Figure 13-4). A wall-mounted machine that easily reaches the patient's mouth where it is positioned for dental procedures should be considered for most practices. This seems to be the most convenient and easy to use. If there are two or more dental procedure tables that a single x-ray machine cannot reach, then consider additional x-ray machines for each location. X-ray machines are relatively inexpensive compared to the value of having a convenient and readily available x-ray source wherever dental procedures are performed.

## Safety

The International Commission on Radiological Protection makes safety recommendations based on justification, optimization, and limitation. *Justification* means exposures should not be done unless a positive net benefit can be expected. *Optimization* mandates using the least amount of radiation required to produce the needed result. And *limitation* speaks to the dose equivalence limits allowed for employees.

Radiopaque areas on a radiograph indicate that the patient's tissues interacted with the x rays, deflecting some but absorbing most. X-rays (similar to gamma rays) are a type of ionizing radiation. Ionization can affect tissues in multiple ways, but the ones of concern during dental radiographs are the somatic stochastic effects; damaging effects that may occur with any dose of radiation. A safe dose has not been possible to determine experimentally. Every exposure carries the possibility of inducing these effects that include leukemia and certain tumors. While a decreased radiation dose reduces the probability of damage occurring, if damage does occur the dose does not affect the severity of the cell damage. It has been estimated that the risk of developing a fatal cancer from two average intraoral dental exposures is around 1:2 million.

Sources of exposure to radiation include the primary beam, scatter radiation, and leakage from the tube head. Leakage should be discovered and resolved during regularly scheduled equipment testing. The radiation emitted when an x-ray is made scatters from the patient in all directions, but a much larger amount passes directly through the patient; it is not blocked. Dental film does not use an intensifying screen. Therefore much larger doses of radiation are needed to expose it than are required for film in cassettes. The quantity of x-rays that pass completely through the patient and exits the other side is far more than is needed for a diagnostic radiograph (Figure 13-5). Staff should minimize their exposure by standing at least 6 feet from the tube head and always at an angle of 90 to 135 degrees from the path of the primary beam. This eliminates the possibility of ever being close to the primary beam and precludes the ability to hold film in position during a radiograph exposure.

Radiation safety procedures must be in place AND must be followed. It is the veterinarian's responsibility to see to this.

Use short-cone technique and either high-speed film or digital radiography to minimize the quantity and energy of x-rays needed to make an image.

## Digital Radiography

Digital radiography refers to computer-generated images of radiographs. Indirect methods of obtaining digital images include either taking a convention radiograph that is then digitized using a data input device or making the exposure on a photostimulatable phosphor plate followed by transferring the latent image to a computer. Direct-to-digital equipment

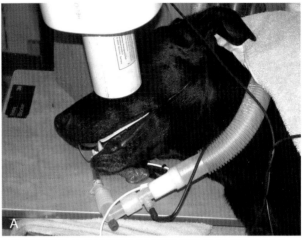
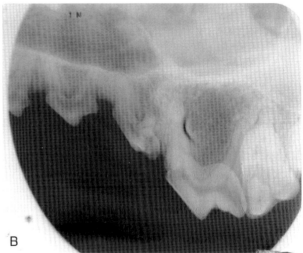
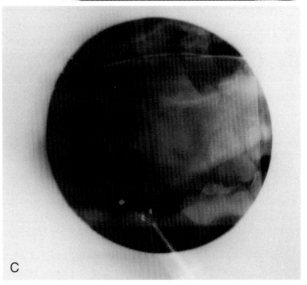

**FIGURE 13-5 Radiation in the primary beam. A,** Patient positioned with a high sensitivity high-speed dental film (size 4 F-speed) positioned for a radiograph of the maxillary fourth premolar tooth. An x-ray cassette with intensifying screens is placed beneath the patient to detect x-rays that pass through the patient. **B,** Diagnostic radiograph made on the dental film. **C,** Even after traveling through the patient and dental film, the exposure on the conventional film was too overexposed to read.

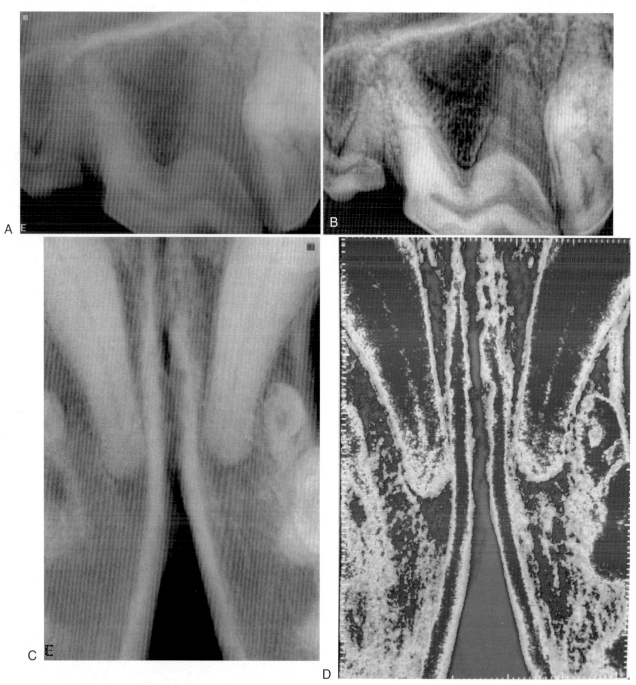

FIGURE 13-6 Digital image enhancement. **A,** Radiograph of a maxillary fourth premolar tooth. **B,** Revealer mode enhances the image. **C,** Radiograph of mandibular canine teeth. **D,** Colorization.

uses either a charge-coupled device (CCD) or a complementary metal oxide semiconductor (CMOS) sensor as a data input device that sends the x-ray image directly to a computer. This is the easiest and most time-efficient method. Most modern x-ray machines are compatible with most digital hardware and software packages. However, before purchasing either a new x-ray machine or a new digital sensor and software system, one should verify that the x-ray machine is capable of short enough exposure times for the digital equipment. Older x-ray machines cannot be used with digital sensors because most digital systems require exposure settings as low as 0.02 second for small patients.

Advantages of direct digital systems include the following:
- Provides immediate image availability
- Eliminates the need for using and disposing of developing and fixing fluids

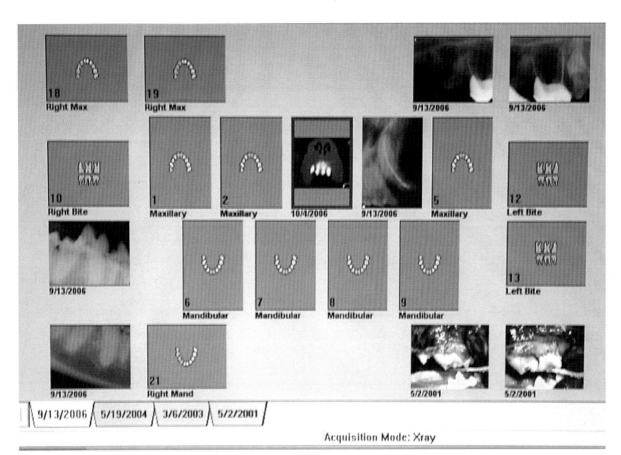

**FIGURE 13-7** Display of digital radiographs and imported images. Note the date tabs on the lower left that correlate to the original procedure (premolar tooth root canal) and follow-up radiographs. On the lower right are imported images of the fractured tooth pretreatment. In the center is an imported image from a CT scan. This image set can be printed for the client.

- Eliminates errors during development
- Allows digital enhancement to assist visualization (Figure 13-6)
- Provides printed visit information for clients
- Automatically labels and stores images referenced to client and patient information (Figure 13-7)
- Requires less radiation
- Templates for referral letters are integrated into most systems

Disadvantages include the following:

- Initial expense
- For some systems, ongoing maintenance and support fees
- Largest sensor size is number 2 (Figures 13-8 and 13-9)

In their practice, the authors have used digital radiography since 1995 and have remained with the original

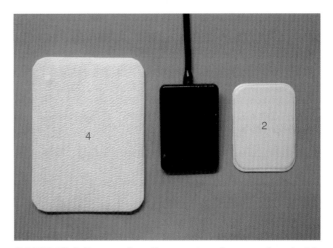

**FIGURE 13-8** Sensor size. The number 2 sensor (center) is similar in size to a size 2 (periapical) emulsion film (marked 2) and much smaller than a number 4 (occlusal) film (marked 4).

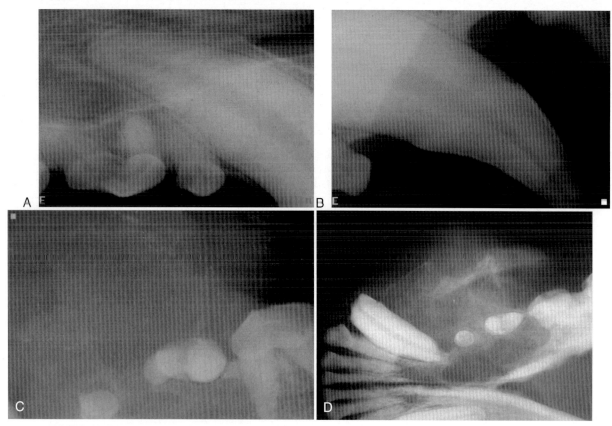

**FIGURE 13-9 Small sensor size. A,** Radiograph of a large canine tooth cannot image the entire tooth. **B,** Second radiograph is required. **C,** Radiograph of a mandibular osteosarcoma is unsatisfactory due to lack of orientation and surrounding structures. **D,** The same tumor radiographed with larger film.

software and hardware with the exception of a sensor up-grade from a CCD to a CMOS. Thirteen years ago, there were only a few manufacturers of digital equipment available. There are currently many from which to choose. Some vendors have been in the business for decades, and more are becoming available on a regular basis. There are some differences in image quality between sensors, and the various software programs offer diverse capabilities and user-friendliness. It would be inappropriate to discuss specific equipment because the field is constantly changing. The size 2 sensor is the only one needed for dogs and cats. The smaller size 1 sensor may be helpful for smaller exotic animals. We look forward to a size 4 sensor becoming available in the future.

## SUGGESTED READINGS

Gibilesco JA: *Stafne's Oral radiographic diagnosis,* Philadelphia, 1985, WB Saunders.

Harvey CE, Emily PP: *Small animal dentistry,* St. Louis, 1993, Mosby.

Whaites E: *Essentials of dental radiography and radiology,* ed 3, New York, 2002, Churchill Livingstone.

Wiggs RB, Lobprise HB: *Veterinary dentistry principles and practice,* Philadelphia, 1997, Lippincott-Raven.